Chén Xiūyuán's 陳修園

金匱方歌括

Formulas from the Golden Cabinet with Songs

Jīn Guì Fāng Gē Kuò

Volumes I - III

Sabine Wilms

The Chinese Medicine Database
www.cm-db.com
Portland, Oregon

Formulas from the Golden Cabinet with Songs

金匱方歌括

Jīn Guì Fāng Gē Kuò

Volume I - III

Sabine Wilms

1017 SW Morrison #306
Portland, OR 97205 USA

COMP designation original Chinese work and English translation

Cover Design by Jonathan Schell L.Ac.
Library of Congress Cataloging-in-Publication Data:

Chen, Xiuyuan, 1753-1823.
[Formulas from the Golden Cabinet with Songs. English]
Jin Gui Fang Ge Kuo = Formulas from the Golden Cabinet with Songs
/ translation Sabine Wilms
p. cm.
Includes Index.
ISBN 978-0-9799552-5-9 (alk. paper)
Medicine, Chinese I. Wilms, Sabine. II. Title: Formulas from the Golden Cabinet with Songs
III. Title: Vol. I - III

International Standard Book Number (ISBN): 978-0-9799552-5-9
Printed in the United States of America

Contents

Appendices

Indices

Chén Niànzǔ, aka Chén Xiūyuán (1753- 1823 CE) was orphaned at young age and lived in poverty. He was adopted by his grandfather and grew up with an extraordinary drive to shake the shackles of his disadvantaged past. He studied the canons as well as medicine and at the age of twenty-four took up the practice of medicine as his profession. But physicians of the time did not enjoy much respect in society and Chén aspired to pursue the path of Zhāng Zhòngjǐng by entering into official government employ. Nevertheless, during his multiple decades working for various counties and agencies throughout Héběi province, he never interrupted his practice of medicine and became well known for saving many a life of both dignitaries as well as commoners alike, resulting him in ultimately becoming as physician and not as an official.

During his years in government service, Chén authored many medical books, of which sixteen have survived the tooth of time, though more are suspected to have been written. As a scholar-clinician, his main interest lay in the study and practice of the *Shānghán Lùn* and *Jīnguì Yàolüè*, and his scholarly endeavors in this field, earned him a spot among the great *Qīng* dynasty *Shānghán Lùn* scholars of the time. Chén studied the *Huángdì Nèijīng* with dedication and even authored a treatise summarizing the essence of both *Sùwèn* and *Língshū*. He also became a representative protagonist of the Phase and Qì *yùnqì* School of *Shānghán Lùn* scholarship, explaining the six conformation theory through the lens of yīn yáng transformation and five phase and six qì dynamics. But he was also a teacher and taught medicine to whoever wanted to learn. It is because of this that he wrote his books with medical songs. Three of these books recorded Formula Songs, which facilitate a student's process of learning and memorization while explaining complex formulas and clinical patterns with great precision and virtuosity. The book you are holding is one of these works, dedicated to explaining the lines of the original texts and summarizing the prescriptions of the *Jīnguì Yàolüè*, allowing for easy reference and facilitating the necessary process of learning by heart.

Today, Chinese medicine practitioners can once more indulge in the graciousness of the hardworking medical sinologist Dr. Sabine Wilms who has again rendered a very necessary translation of an important scholarly and clinically relevant work. The resultant translation of the *Jīn Guì Fāng Gē Kuò* is very accessible to aspiring herbalists while being uncompromising in depth and quality of discourse. As an avid *Shānghán Lùn* clinician, I am thrilled by what will hopefully become a trend of translating previously unavailable antique *Shānghán* and *Jīnguì* commentaries from the *Míng* and *Qīng* dynasties, allowing non-Chinese reading acupuncturists and herbalists alike greater access to these highly practical gems of Chinese medicine scholarship.

Arnaud Versluys, PhD, MD (China), LAc
Institute of Classics in East Asian Medicine
Portland, OR, USA

Publisher's Note

1) The focus of the Chinese Medicine Database is on the translation of the classical texts of Chinese medicine. While this statement seems self-evident, there is some confusion as to what this means. If we talk about the classical texts as source material for the field of Chinese medicine, then we are concerned with translating the source material.

Translation, though, does not always mean commentary or analysis. As a field we have a choice about how to use our scholarly resources. The numbers of people who are qualified to translate Chinese medical texts into acceptable English are actually very few. Not all of these people are Chinese medicine professionals. Some are sinologists and some are historians. The Database sees translation as similar to gathering data. In any medical study, there are several phases, generally in this order: the rules of the study are created, participants are selected, the data is gathered, the data is analyzed, and lastly a report is generated.

For us, the rules of the study are the use of a consistent terminology throughout our publications. Participants are the texts that we translate. Gathering of data is translation of the source texts. Data analysis is commentary by doctoral students, qualified professionals, and scholars. Lastly, report generation is the consensus that is reached in our field on any source text.

The Database sees itself as just one part in this process. You, the reader, are also part of this process. In 1979 Dr. Hong-Yen Hsu, Ph.D., wrote in the preface to his book *Treating Cancer with Chinese Herbs*[1]:

> "The Oriental Healing Arts Institute was founded to collect and make available to the Western world translations of all the major classical and contemporary works on Chinese medicine .... By making this information available we hope to stimulate interest in the Chinese medical legacy so that further research will be done in the West."

This was 31 years ago, and I ask you, how far have we come since this mission statement was written? Hence the Database has made the hard decision to focus on the pure translation of these texts. Some have reviewed our texts and wished that they had more commentary, and I agree that often the meaning of these old texts is obscure and esoteric, but where as a field should we start? One cannot write books without touching pen to paper, as the saying goes, and so too as a field we can not begin to have public discourse about the classics of Chinese medicine without being able to

1. Oriental Healing Arts Institute, 1990, p. xiii.

read them in our native language.

If the Database can provide interested practitioners with a window into these old texts, then in my opinion we have fulfilled our mission. Your part is to analyze the data in these old texts and see what you believe and what you don't believe. Assimilate the parts that work for you and throw out the rest, but at least our texts provide you with an entire book, so that you the reader can follow the original author's train of thought. Hopefully from this content you will find insights into Chinese medicine and life that resonate with your practice.

2) We have left the Chinese measurements in the running text, but in the translation we have changed the measurements into grams and milliliters to make the text more accessible to practitioners.

It seems that there are two different schools of thought as to the translation of measurements from Chinese into English. We have followed our previous translation of the *Bei Ji Qian Jin Yao Fang* as well as Huang Huang's conversions in his book *Zhang Zhongjing's Clinical Applications of 50 Medicinals.*[2] The conversions are as follows:

Volume:

5 dǒu	斗	=	1 hú	斛	=	10 liters
10 shēng	升	=	1 dǒu	斗	=	2 liters
10 gě	合	=	1 shēng	升	=	200ml
			1 gě	合	=	20ml

Weight:

1 jīn	斤	48g
1 liǎng	兩	3g
1 qián	錢	0.3g
1 fēn	分	0.75g

There is another school of thought on conversion, though, and I have heard enough herbalists talk about this conversion strategy that I believe it warrants including. It is only in reference to weight:

1 jīn	斤	480g
1 liǎng	兩	30g

2. People's Medical Publishing House, 2008, p. 561

1 qián	錢	3g
1 fēn	分	0.3g

Obviously, these are quite significant differences in dosage. In the end, formulas come down to ratios and one's own understanding as an herbalist of how herb dosing is effective. We have chosen the path of the minimalist. If you believe in larger doses in your practice, then all you need to do is multiply our measurements in the text by ten, and you will arrive at this second dosing strategy.

We believe that presenting the dosage in grams and milliliters will save the practitioner time when adopting these valuable formulas in your clinical practice.

Jonathan Schell L.Ac.
The Chinese Medicine Database
Portland, OR
November, 4, 2010

Translator's Preface

Whether we as translators are honest enough to admit it or not, the act of translation invariably involves making hard choices that reflect the translator's academic and clinical background as well as his or her personal preferences. To name just a few issues that my publisher and I have spent months in heated discussion over in our effort to make Zhāng Zhòngjǐng's and Chén Xiūyuán's pearls of wisdom accessible to modern clinical readers, we have struggled with terminology, presentation and formatting, conversion of measurements, interpretative notes, and explanation of concepts that are ultimately unexplainable in a different medical and cosmological paradigm. This holds particularly true in a text from a culture so far removed from our modern Euro-American context as historical Chinese medical literature. And to make matters even worse, the present translation concerns an early nineteenth century commentary on a late second or early third century text that even the commentator had questions about.

In the following paragraphs, I briefly address a few of these issues to illustrate to the reader where I am coming from in my own work and why I choose to translate and write the way I do. I realize that there are no perfect solutions and that all approaches have their advantages and disadvantages. The field of Chinese medical literature in translation is still in its infancy and the process of forming a consensus is always painful and drawn-out. My academic training as a historian, medical anthropologist, and sinologist predisposes me to what some practitioners may consider an extreme commitment to preservation, as opposed to interpretation, of the source. As a result, I create literal translations that force modern readers -- along with me -- to occasionally stumble and shake their heads in confusion, rather than handing them a neatly explained package. In my eyes, complicated passages that have caused headaches to thousands of Chinese scholars and physicians for almost two millennia deserve and need to be preserved as such, rather than being simplified into one translator's personal understanding and modern clinical interpretation.

I realize and openly admit that my reading of certain passages is shaky - to me, that is the beauty of classical Chinese literature; that is where the art of Chinese medicine begins; and that is also an essential requirement if we are to be honest as a profession about the difficulty of practicing a medicine from a vastly different cultural context. On a personal level, I read the early medical classics not only as clinical information but also as philosophical ruminations, as expressions of their authors' insights into the nature of the cosmos and our human existence within it. I treat them as divinely inspired wisdom that will not reveal itself to anybody in a cursory reading but over a lifetime of study and experience. Because of this attitude, pinning my current understanding down on paper in a published English translation is a difficult process, one that opens me up to easy criticism from people who disagree with me for many reasons, valid and informed or not. Nevertheless, I feel strongly enough about the importance of this material that I see the need to open up this world to practitioners and students who are unable to read the classics in the original classical Chinese, without inserting my by necessity limited interpretation of the material into the source. English readers have a right to direct access to the sources, unmediated (as much as humanly possible) by the translator's understanding thereof. My caveat here would be that the classics cannot be fully grasped in depth by just reading them in English but must be discussed with peers, contemplated, experienced in clinic, revised, and reread over and over. It is my hope that this book will facilitate this process!

Many times over the past years, I have been tempted to follow Lǎozǐ's example and ride away on an ox into the mountains because the contemporary English language, being a creation of the modern human mind, is simply inadequate for conveying complex and essential medical concepts like *xū* 虛 and *shí* 實: As any informed reader is aware of, this most basic pair of terms is usually translated in the medical context either as "vacuity" and "repletion" (Wiseman/Paradigm and Blue Poppy) or as "depletion" and "excess" (Eastland) respectively. Literally and in their common use in Chinese, the characters simply mean "empty/hollow" (in the sense of an absence or lack of something) and "full" (in the sense of "solid," illustrated by the pictograph, which depicts a string of cash under a roof). If either vacuity/repletion or depletion/excess were perfect translations, this debate would have been settled a long time ago. Many practitioners find "vacuity" and "repletion" offensive and unnecessarily stilted for such fundamental concepts, which they have to communicate to their patients on a daily basis. Choosing them unequivocally places you in the "Wiseman camp" and presumably makes your work inaccessible to scores of readers who simply don't have the stomach for awkward and hair-splitting terminological issues. After giving "excess" and "deficiency" an honest try in a large number of contexts in this text, I have chosen to return to Wiseman terminology for the simple reason that it more accurately conveys the meaning of the Chinese terms and that I find "excess" and "deficiency" to be unacceptably misleading for what they mean in the common English language.

For the same reason, I strictly adhere to Wiseman terminology throughout this book, with a handful of exceptions that I have noted in the footnotes. I continue to use the terminology explained in the *Practical Dictionary of Chinese Medicine* by Nigel Wiseman and Feng Ye (Paradigm Publications, 1998) for two simple reasons: First, I have found it to reflect the authors' deep commitment to conveying the meaning of Chinese medicine in its historical and cultural context rather than translating it into modern biomedical terms. Second, this dictionary presents the only consistent reference base for the technical terminology in Chinese medicine. Allowing readers to know the precise Chinese equivalent for any English term, the *Dictionary* in addition provides succinct explanations that are both historically and culturally sensitive and clinically relevant.

On a more general note, a few sentences are in order on the selection of this text and the format the Chinese Medicine Database and I created for presenting it in this book. My fascination with Zhāng

Zhòngjǐng's *Jīn Guì Yào Lüè* started many years ago, when I had the honor of working with my friend and mentor Nigel Wiseman on a manuscript translation of this text for Paradigm Publications. Like hosts of practitioners, teachers, and students of Chinese medicine, I have been waiting for the long over-due publication of this essential early classical text. Being aware of its clinical significance, it did not take much convincing when Jonathan Schell approached me last year with the request to translate the present book with Chén Xiūyuán's commentary. An enlightened scholar, dedicated and skilled physician, and prolific author, Chén Xiūyuán created an impressive body of medical literature based on his profound understanding of the classics. Inspired by decades of clinical experience paired with his broad erudition and family tradition of practicing as enlightened scholar-physicians, Chén devoted much to making the treasures of classical Chinese medicine accessible to people less fortunate or educated than himself.

As the present book will hopefully show, these efforts continue to bear fruit to this day. Chén's work deserves to be fully accessible to all students of Chinese medicine, whether they can read classical Chinese or not. This book is the beginning of what we envision one day to become a complete set of translations of Chén's work. Given the length of his commentary on the *Jīn Guì Yào Lüè*, we have decided to divide the original six scrolls of the *Jīn Guì Fāng Gē Kuò* into two books, of which the present book is the first half.

Because no complete literal English translation of this important source text exists as of yet in English, we have added the full text for formulas from the original *Jīn Guì Yào Lüè*, wherever it was missing from Chén Xiūyuán's commentary. While Zhang Zhòngjǐng's formulas and explanations thereof were apparently sufficiently known to Chén's original readers that he did not feel the need to give the full text of the source in each instance, the same is unfortunately not true for our modern readership. By supplementing missing text from the *Jīn Guì Yào Lüè*, we have made sure that this book can be read as a stand-alone text, rather than requiring a copy of the *Jīn Guì Yào Lüè* to read alongside it.

Lastly, to further increase the applicability of this material in the modern clinical context, we have added a formula appendix for quick reference. This appendix is composed of translated excerpts from the formula entries in an early twentieth century edition of the *Zhōng Guó Yī Xué Dà Cí Diǎn* 中國醫學大辭典 (*Great Dictionary of Medicine in China*). To facilitate easy referencing, we have chosen to abbreviate the entries to include only the formula name, ingredients and amounts, major indications, and a summary of the formula analysis. This appendix contains information on all the formulas mentioned in the *Jīn Guì Yào Lüè*.

Sabine Wilms,
Taos, New Mexico,
November 1, 2010.

Acknowledgments

In the past decades, our modern understanding of classical Chinese medicine has continued to deepen, progress, and evolve in response to the modern clinical context and the challenges of our times. I am firmly convinced that the medical and cosmological wisdom expressed in these ancient Chinese classics can play a significant part in the ongoing and universal human effort to heal bodies and minds in a rapidly changing world. I hope this book can be a small contribution.

Creating a translation of a classical medical text with no outside funding is by definition a labor of love. It would have never happened without the cooperation of my daughter Momo, who helped with milking goats, processing apples, cooking dinners, raising chicks, and countless other farm chores. Thanks for making me stop my brain and eat, sleep, wrestle dogs, feel the sunshine, and savor the every-day miracles of our farming adventure and life together!

Writing books while raising a kid and running a farm requires many many hands besides my own. I am grateful to my friends Sandra Gonzales and Tomas Martinez for having lent much-needed support and encouragement, and to Autumn Bitterlich and various other goat milkers and farm sitters for holding up the fort while I was away attending conferences or giving lectures. I obviously couldn't have done it without you!

I am also deeply indebted to the criticism, questions, and suggestions from a large number of practitioner friends, colleagues, readers, and participants in my various courses who have had to suffer through countless discussions on translation issues. Besides giving me invaluable feedback on the clinical significance of the material I translate, though, they have also helped me to crystallize my understanding of and appreciation for early Chinese medicine in general. The longer and more deeply I become involved with this material, the more certain I grow of its importance, on both a clinical and a personal level. Having to explain the importance of the classics to busy modern practitioners who just want to know "where to stick the needle" has been a challenge that has forced me to formulate a good answer in my head, one that grows stronger and stronger each time I have to give it. I so appreciate all the schools, conference organizers, and teachers who share my commitment to teaching the classical foundations of Chinese medicine. And of course I am grateful for the host of enthusiastic listeners whose intellectual curiosity forces me to keep going and add yet another 10 texts to my list of future projects every day.

While my Chinese medicine consultants are too many to list here, I need to give special credit to Lorraine Wilcox and Henry McCann who graciously read the entire manuscript and gave many

many valuable comments. I am also grateful to Z'ev Rosenberg for his steady support and feedback; to Arnaud Versluys for writing a preface and tirelessly promoting the importance of Zhāng Zhòngjǐng's work in his own teaching; to John Moffett for speedily supplying us with copies of the source texts when needed; and to my publisher Jonathan Schell for the months of heated discussions while we were trying to strike a balance between making this material clinically applicable and yet staying truthful to the historical source. A large debt of gratitude is owed to Nigel Wiseman who started my love for the *Jīn Guì* so many years back, when I had the honor of working with him on the original text. Lastly, thanks go to my favorite acupuncturist and Qigong teacher Jim Dixon for inspiring me to practice!

This book is dedicated to all the peace makers of the world, the parents and teachers and caretakers and healers who spread their love and joy and grace around as the sun rises each day. It is my sincere hope that my translations of classical Chinese medicine will inspire you and open your eyes not only to a beautiful and efficacious medical paradigm, but also to a cosmology, to a vision of harmonious and balanced existence in the social, natural, and cosmic web of existence that our present world has great need for.

Sabine Wilms,
Taos, New Mexico,
November 1, 2010.

Introduction by Yaron Seidman

Chén Xiūyuán 陳修園, a famous Chinese medicine scholar from the *Qīng* 清 dynasty, was born in the eighteenth year of the Qián Lóng 乾隆 reign period (i.e., 1753) in Fújiàn 福建 province, Chánglè 長樂 county, in the village of Xīméi 溪眉 in the town of Jiāngtiān 江天. He died in the third year of the Dào Guāng 道光 reign period (i.e. 1823) in the city of Róng Chěng 榕城 (today's Fúzhōu 福州 in Fújiàn 福建 province). His birth name (*míng* 名) was Chén Niànzǔ 陳念祖 and his given name as an adult (*zì* 字) was Chén Xiūyuán 陳修園. He also adopted the pen names (*hào* 號) Liángyǒu 良有 and Shènxiū 慎修, by which he was known best during his lifetime. He lived to be 71 years old.

Chén Xiūyuán's life

According to his historical biography, Xiūyuán lost his father early in life, and his family was poverty-stricken. He was raised and educated by his grandfather Chén Jūláng 陳居郎 who was a master of medicine himself. Having started memorizing classical texts at the tender age of seven, Xiūyuán already finished studying the Confucian classics and started his study of medicine at the age of fourteen. In those days, medicine was viewed as a socially inferior occupation and Xiūyuán therefore decided to pursue an official position in government in addition to medicine, to change his life circumstances.

At the age of nineteen, he passed the imperial examination at the county level, attaining the degree of *xiùcái* 秀才, and one year later started practicing medicine in his hometown in order to help people, as well as teaching pupils. Soon thereafter, he left home to pursue advanced studies at the prestigious Áo Fēng Academy 鰲峰書院 in Fúzhōu, where he studied the Confucian and historical classics in depth under Mèng Chāorán 孟超然. At this time, Chén's studies of medicine had deepened considerably and he started writing his first book, titled *Shāng hán lùn qiǎn zhù* 傷寒論淺注 (*Shallow Commentary on the Shāng Hán Lùn*), which he completed in 1796.

In 1792, he passed the imperial exam at the provincial level, attaining the degree of *zhòngjǔ* 中舉, and went north to Běijīng to take the imperial exam. After failing to pass this examination, he remained in Běijīng for an extended period of time to practice medicine. At this time, a famous government official named Yī Cháodòng 伊朝棟 suffered a stroke, for which no doctor could help him. Chén prescribed a potent formula and his illustrious patient soon recovered. From this point on, his name became famous throughout the capital. A famous *Qīng* minister of defense contracted a grave disease of feet atrophy, which Chén was able to cure. This minister subsequently tried to convince Chén to become his personal physician and offered him a post at the imperial medical college, which Chén, however, firmly declined under the pretense of sickness. He then returned to his family home in Chánglè to serve as the principal of Wú Háng Academy 吳航書院, where he taught the Confucian and medical classics. After two years, he moved to Quánzhōu 泉州 to lecture at the Qīng Yuán Academy 清源書院 where he also studied under the famous doctor Cài Zōngyù 蔡宗玉.

In the year 1800, he returned to the capital to take the highest exam and was, after successful graduation, dispatched by the emperor to Bǎoyāng 保陽. The following year he became a county magistrate in Wēi 威 county. At this time, he participated in an imperial relief effort in response to catastrophic rains in the North of China and was later promoted to the position of Prefectural Chief (*zhīzhōu* 知州). On one occasion, he acted as an agent of the prefecture's magistrate. In all his official duties, Master Chén was known to be a noble and virtuous official who helped the common people. For example, in 1801 he learned that in Wēi county many women were suffering from uterine prolapse. On their behalf, he ordered the manufacture of special internal and external prescriptions, which resulted in the cure and recovery of many. On another occasion, torrential rains affected the area around Héng Shān 恆山 mountain and he resolved to inspect the disaster area himself. He discovered that malaria was raging among the people and that many doctors were treating it erroneously, resulting in many deaths. He thus ordered the manufacture of three different pills addressing three different syndromes. He instructed the population in how to differentiate between the three syndromes and how to administer the correct pills. The pills were widely distributed, resulting in a cure for many. In his spare time he collected 108 prescription poems and sent them to press. These helped instruct many doctors in how to achieve a good cure for their patients. Many lives were saved as a result.

In 1802, the governor-general of Zhílì 直隸 province (today's Héběi 河北), suffered a stroke. Master Chén prescribed *Huáng Qí Wǔ Wù Tāng* 黄芪五物湯 (Astragalus Five Substance Decoction), to be taken regularly, and combined it with pills that supplemented the kidneys and liver, which resulted in a cure. Subsequently, he was praised highly by the governor-general. Around the same time he published the *Jǐng Yuè Xīn Fāng Biān* 景岳新方砭 (*Critique of Jǐngyuè's New Prescriptions*). Later that year, when his mother fell ill and died, he returned to his family home. At that time, he published two other books: *Shí Fāng Miào Yòng* 時方妙用 (*Marvelous Effect of Modern Prescriptions*) and *Shí Fāng Gē Kuò* 時方歌括 (*Modern Prescriptions with Poems*). In addition, two other books, *Yī Xué Sān Zì Jīng* 醫學三字經 (*Three-Character Classic of Medicine*) and *Shén Nóng Běn Cǎo Jīng Dú* 神農本草經讀 (*Reading the Divine Farmer's Classic of Materia Medica*) were published in Róng Chěng (Fúzhōu).

In 1808 Xiūyuán went back to the capital to hold office. In his spare time, he composed a new commentary on the *Shāng Hán Lùn* 傷寒論 in rhymed form and compiled the book *Cháng Shā Fāng Gē Kuò* 長沙方歌括 (*Prescriptions from Cháng Shā with Poems*). In order to correct the failing medicine of poor doctors, he also compiled a text called *Yī Xué Shí Zài Yì* 醫學實在易 (*The Study of Medicine is Indeed Easy*).

One example of Chén's superior diagnostic skills is an incident that took place in 1810. An official from Tiān Jīn 天津, came to visit Chén. When Chén saw that his complexion was dark and swollen and that his nose was slightly greenish, he immediately told him that he was suffering from water retention disease that involved the liver. According to Chén, if treated immediately there could be a cure, but if not treated within the next twenty days it would be too late. The official didn't believe Chén's proclamation, and, twenty days later, fell incurably ill. Even Chén's efforts at that point could not save the man.

In 1819 Chén had enough of political life and retired back to Fújiàn. Many scholars from all across the country came to study with him. He instructed students systematically and tirelessly in the classics. Throughout his life, Chén compiled medical works that served to improve the quality of medicine practiced by all doctors, and thus to benefit all of humankind. In 1823 he fell ill and subsequently died in Róng Chěng at the age of 71. His body was returned to his hometown in the village of Xīméi for burial.

Chén's children and grandchildren carried on his art and further arranged his books: These include his eldest son Chén Yuánbào 陳元豹 and second son Chén Yuánxī 陳元犀. Chén Yuánbào's sons were Chén Zhūzhì 陳諸治, Chén Zhūqiào 陳諸翹, and Chén Zhūdé 陳諸德. Chén Yuánxī's sons were Chén Xīndiǎn 陳心典 and Chén Xīnlán 陳心蘭. Several of the prefaces to Chén Xiūyuán's books contain the signature of Chén Xīndiǎn as the eldest grandson, testifying that Chén Zhūzhì possibly died at an early age and that Chén Yuánxī's eldest son was the leading figure in arranging and compiling the texts and commentaries of his father and grandfather.

Chén Xiūyuán's Accomplishments

Even though Chén Xiūyuán served as an official for many years, his ultimate contribution to society was his dedication to medicine and the medical classics. In the study of medicine he was influenced by Zhāng Zhìcōng 張志聰 and Gāo Shìzōng 高士宗 and their commentaries of the ancient classics. In his book *Yī Xué Sān Zì Jīng*, he writes that, "The great authors are from Qián Táng 錢塘." This is the name of a river in Zhèjiāng 浙江 province, where both Zhāng and Gāo lived. He believed that Wáng Shūhé arranged the *Shāng Hán Lùn* in a truthful manner and disputed scholars who claimed that the original text was altered by Wáng. He was often referred to as the scholar who believes in the ancient ways. However, like the predecessors, teachers, and scholars who inspired him, he too was on the quest for truth. The ancient classics were the path toward seeking this truth. In his argument and criticism of other scholars like Zhāng Jǐngyuè 張景岳, Lǐ Shízhēn 李時珍, and Lǐ Gǎo 李杲, he often agreed with their accomplishments but disagreed with what he believed to be their departure from the truth of the sages. For example, he said that Lǐ Gǎo was biased towards supplementation of the spleen and stomach but that his methods were nevertheless useful and accurate as the spleen and stomach were indeed very important. He was very critical of Lǐ Shízhēn's masterpiece, the *Běn Cǎo Gāng Mù* 本草綱目 (*Systematic Materia Medica*) yet considered his writing on the pulse *Bīn Hú Mài Xué* 瀕湖脈學 (*Study of the Pulse on the Lakeside*) as most superior. He sharply criticized Zhāng Jǐngyuè in his book *Jǐng Yuè Xīn Fāng Biān*, yet used his formula *Liù Ān Jiān* 六安煎 [Six Pacifiers Brew] as the first formula for cough from cold damage in his book *Yī Xué Sān Zì Jīng*. He systematically analyzed Jǐngyuè's book, which despite his criticism meant that he studied it well. Among 186 new prescriptions in Jǐngyuè's book, Chén concluded that 20 were superior, 60 entirely inadequate, and only 80 were average. Chén was a great believer in the medicine and classics before the *Hàn* and *Táng* dynasties, yet he also studied the accomplished masters of the *Jīn*, *Yuán*, *Míng* and *Qīng* dynasties up to his time. He believed that one must find the strong points of each and follow them, and find the bad aspects of each and discard them.

During Chén's lifetime most doctors would study medical texts from the *Sòng*, *Jīn*, and *Yuán* dynasties and neglect to study the ancient classics. He explained that doctors don't understand the *Dào* 道 ["Way"] of medicine because they fail to thoroughly research the classics. As such his lifetime pursuit was the knowledge of the classics, namely the *Nèijīng*, *Nàn Jīng*, *Shāng Hán Lùn*, *Jīn Guì Yào Lüè*, *Shén Nóng Běn Cǎo Jīng*, and the Confucian classics. As he explained in his *Yī Xué Sān Zì Jīng*:

> If the principles are not based on the *Nèijīng* and the applications of Zhòngjǐng's methods are well mastered, then even though you may get lucky once, you cannot attain the true principles.

Chén was aware that many doctors had lost the old ways of medicine, so he dedicated his life to researching the old ways and explaining their difficult concepts in plain words. Many doctors all across China, with no proper education, studied medicine from Chén Xiūyuán's books and later became famous physicians. His sixteen books were widely sold all across China. Because of their later popularity, he accumulated texts from other writers, some known and some unknown, to create new compilations under his name such as: Chén Xiūyuán's eighteen books, twenty-one books, twenty-four books, thirty-two books, forty-eight books and even seventy-two books. His legacy among the medicial sages of China is due to his "shallow commentaries" on the *Nèijīng*, *Shāng Hán Lùn* and *Jīn Guì Yào Lüè*. In an era where the ancient classics were long forgotten because of their abstract and hard to comprehend language, he simplified comprehension by inserting his commentary in between the lines of the ancient texts. His commentary made the texts easier to understand and gave confidence to his reader that they could comprehend the difficult concepts in the ancient texts. This in turn led to a significant trend of rediscovering the classics. Following Zhāng Zhìcōng's lead in the revival of the classics, Chén Xiūyuán stands out in the history of Chinese medicine as a figure that revived the medical classics throughout the entire country and to an extent with an entire generation.

Research Into the Medical Classics

Chén Xiūyuán viewed the *Nèijīng* as the core of Chinese medicine. Without thorough research into it, one cannot advance to studying herbs and formulas, nor can one understand the *Shāng Hán Lùn* and *Jīn Guì Yào Lüè*. He realized that in any given place of the ancient text a discussion of a certain difficulty is not a stand-alone discussion and that the same difficulty may appear in other places in the text from a different perspective. In his research into the *Nèijīng*, he used a method of "categorization," already used by other scholars like Zhāng Jǐngyuè, which brought related arguments of the same subject under one roof. In this way different aspects of the same difficulty could be considered and analyzed simultaneously, resulting in a deeper understanding by the student. Nevertheless, this style of learning by means of categorization historically had two schools. One school, lead by scholars like Zhāng Jǐngyuè and Yáng Shàngshàn 楊上善, believed that the entire text of the *Nèijīng* must be preserved and categorized from beginning to end. The other school, presented by scholars like Lǐ Zhōngzǐ 李中梓 and Wāng Áng 汪昂, believed that only certain parts of the *Nèijīng* needed or should be categorized together. Chén Xiūyuán followed the second school, categorizing only parts of the text and not its entirety. He selected certain "essential sections" (*jié yào* 節要), in order to compose his *Nèijīng* commentary. Regarding Chén's interpretation of the *Nèijīng*, his special contribution is his commentary to the theory of *Yùn Qì* 運氣 or the transformations of heavenly energy and their impact on the human body, health, and disease. The seven chapters of the *Nèijīng* that deal with this subject come from distant antiquity and the language is particularly difficult to understand. Chén's commentary in using plain language greatly impacted and inspired the Chinese medicine community, as it allowed access to this ancient and previously hard to decipher knowledge.

As for the *Shāng Hán Lùn*, Chén opposed the notion that the original text was altered by Wáng Shūhé, as some suggested. Like Zhāng Zhìcōng, he felt that the text from beginning to end had a logical link suggesting that the entire work was original. Chén did believe that a few segments were added by Wáng, but only to clarify and expand on the master's original meaning and not, as others believed, "to create chaos" in the text. In his own words in the *Shāng Hán Lùn Qiǎn Zhù* 傷寒論淺注 (*Shallow Commentary on Shāng Hán Lùn*) he states:

> Zhòngjǐng is like Confucius in the Confucian school, and Wáng Shūhé is like Confucius' disciple Zǐ Xià 子夏, who could not argue with the master...

Therefore, he could not have inserted additional segments into the original text under his own name and hence merely continued his master's words. In his research of the *Shāng Hán Lùn*, Chén believed that earlier commentators were lacking in their understanding of the *Shāng Hán Lùn* and that only Zhāng Zhìcōng and Zhāng Lìngsháo 張令韶 were following closely in Zhòngjǐng's steps. In his *Shāng Hán Lùn Qiǎn Zhù*, Chén states:

> Only Zhāng Zhìcōng and Zhāng Lìngsháo have followed the original text in their commentary, even though at times we find a slight crookedness. Yet their elaborations on the five transitions and six qì (*wǔ yùn liù qì* 五運六氣) and on the principle of yīn-yáng joining into one whole conform exactly to Zhòngjǐng's statement in the original preface that he himself used the nine scrolls of the *Sù Wèn* and the *Yīn Yáng Dà Lùn* 陰陽大論 (*Great Discussion on Yīn and Yáng*) [as the sources for his book]. I most admire them. I myself have used the segments from these two commentators in the present book as the core and have added my own commentary in small print.

Chén was a master of the Confucian classics and the ancient arts. His level of accomplishment is seen in the prose of his poems. For example, the *Cháng Shā Fāng Gē Kuò* 長沙方歌括 (*Collection of Prescription Poems from Cháng Shā*) includes the following seven words poem:

> Fresh *fù* [aconite] one piece, one *liǎng jiāng* [ginger], for agitation and vexation during the day with peace all night long, a faint pulse, not outside body no heat, suffering does not stop completely until sunset.

In this four sentence poem, Chén uses the formula *Gān Jiāng Fù Zǐ Tāng* 乾薑附子湯 (Dried Ginger and Aconite Decoction) and explains the ingredients, quantity, symptoms, and application in a rhyming and easy to memorize poem. Even without reading the Chinese, we can see here the mastery of the classical poetry style which Chén had accomplished. Not only was he versed in the *Nèijīng* and *Shāng Hán Lùn*, but also in the traditional way of thinking. For him putting the essence of the ancient classics into rhymed poetry meant the ability to transmit this valuable knowledge to the masses as easily memorized poems, to provide an easy way to study and memorize the classics. And so he composed several of his books in poetry.

Even though Chén was an adherent of the classics and the old ways, in his research of the *Nèijīng* and *Shāng Hán Lùn* he often incorporated new ideas, discoveries, and developments. For example, his commentaries in small print in between the lines expressed innovations that made the original text and commentary flow as one whole, yet the reader could still clearly see the difference between the commentary and the original text. Many of his new ideas are explained in his small print. For example, in a summarizing sentence on *tàiyáng* 太陽 disease, he distinguishes between channel disease and qì disease. In order to explain the disease mechanism, he uses the concepts of root, manifestation, and qì seen from the center (*běn biāo zhōng jiàn zhī qì* 本標中見之氣) as well as that of the opening, closing, and pivot. He explains that in the method of six-spheres diagnosis according to the *Shāng Hán Lùn*, one distinguishes in the three yáng between channel and organ patterns, while the three yīn spheres are differentiated by the transformations of yīn and yáng patterns. In a practical way, he explained the application of these differentiations in clinic. Even though in comparison with other commentators Chén's commentary might be considered less conclusive, it is apparent that the essence of the *Shāng Hán Lùn* is at hand. His development of Zhòngjǐng's diagnostic methods is seen in the *Yī Xué Sān Zì Jīng*:

> "*Cháng Shā* Treatise, (one) sighs at its lofty solidness, preserve essential fluids, its true meaning!"

"*Cháng Shā* Treatise" is the *Shāng Hán Lùn*, which is described as lofty and solid. Chén himself explains that "preserve essential fluids" means that one who is truly skilled at learning can read between the lines, and that this is the true meaning of the classic.

In the *Líng Sù Jié Yào Qiǎn Zhù* 靈素節要淺注 (*Shallow Commentary on Essential Segments of the Líng Sù*), Chén discussed the *Sù Wèn* chapter *Liù Wēi Zhǐ Dà Lùn* 六微旨大論 [Great Treatise on the Six Subtleties], which elucidates that the six qì control each other first and that birth and transformation follow afterwards. The five phases have engendering, transformative, restrictive, and controlling relationships. If there is lack of control, adverse energy arises and causes damage, but if control and restriction exist, there can be transformation and birth.

His Work

Chén composed sixteen books in his lifetime. The following is a chronological narration of his life's work.

1. *Shāng Hán Lùn Qiǎn Zhù* 傷寒論淺注 (*Shallow Commentary on the Shāng Hán Lùn*): ca. 1796 in six scrolls. Chén followed Zhāng Zhìcōng and Zhāng Xījū's 張錫駒 arrangement and commentary. He inserted his commentary in small sized characters in the midst of the original text, allowing an uninterrupted reading of the text in conjunction with his commentary. Chén recognized that each segment contained a method of treatment. Therefore, at the end of each segment, he pointed out what the method was. In his commentary language, he used guiding words and a summary. These features allow the reader a clearer understanding of the text and invoke a desire to study further. His usage of the title "shallow commentary" adds to this momentum as well.

2. *Shí Fāng Gē Kuò* 時方歌括 (*Modern Prescriptions with Poems*): ca. 1801 in two scrolls. A collection of 108 prescriptions from the *Táng* and *Sòng* dynasties, which are divided into twelve categories: supplementing to support weakness, heaviness to calm fear, lightness to expels fullness, expanding to resolve congestion, penetrating to move stagnation, draining to resolve blockages, moistening to solve stiffness, acridity to solidify separation, dampness to moistens dryness, dryness to dispel dampness, cold to overcome heat, and heat to control cold. Each prescription entry

includes the ingredients, main indication, medicinal principle, and modifications. The language is concise and clear to understand, and also includes poetry that is easy to memorize.

3. *Jǐng Yuè Xīn Fāng Biān* 景岳新方砭 (*A Critique of Jǐngyuè's New Prescriptions*): ca. 1802 in four scrolls. Chén took Zhāng Jǐngyuè's newly invented 186 prescriptions and divided them into eight categories: supplementing, harmonizing, attacking, dispersing, cooling, warming, solidifying, and leading. In this book Chén used his knowledge of the classics on formula preparation, medicinal combination, pattern differentiation, etc, to assess and criticize Jǐngyuè's formulas and offer his own advice.

4. *Shén Nóng Běn Cǎo Jīng Dú* 神農本草經讀 (*Reading the Divine Farmer's Classic of Materia Medica*): ca. 1803 in four scrolls. Chén selected 160 commonly used herbs from the ancient materia medica. Subsequent to the commentary by Zhāng Zhìcōng and Yè Guì 葉桂, he added his own discoveries in the spirit of the *Nèijīng* and *Shāng Hán Lùn*.

5. *Shí Fāng Miào Yòng* 時方妙用 (*The Marvelous Effect of Modern Prescriptions*): ca. 1803 in four scrolls. In the first scroll, Chén elaborates on the four diagnostic methods (seeing, hearing, asking, and palpating), and also includes a discussion of stroke and tuberculosis. In scrolls two through four he discusses forty-two commonly occurring diseases and their pathology, symptoms, and treatment principles. It is a practical book that explains the clinical application of medicine.

6. *Yī Xué Sān Zì Jīng* 醫學三字經 (*Three Character Classic of Medicine*): ca. 1804 in four scrolls. The entire book uses poems with lines of three characters, a format that allows the student to easily memorize and appreciate the content. In scrolls one and two, Chén describes the origin of medicine, basic concepts, and symptoms, diagnosis, and treatment of commonly seen ailments. In scrolls three and four he describes in greater detail medicinal prescriptions and their applications, including preparation, modifications, and the theory behind them. In scroll four he also discusses the notions of yīn yáng, *zàng fǔ* (臟腑), and the four diagnostic methods. The language is concise and the poetic language admirable. This book has been reprinted about thirty times in the past 200 years, on average about once every six or seven years. The number of copies printed cannot be matched by any other contemporary author and its influence on doctors of Chinese medicine in the recent era is immense.

7. *Cháng Shā Fāng Gē Kuò* 長沙方歌括 (*Prescriptions from Cháng Shā with Poems*): ca. 1808 in six scrolls. Chén collected 112 *Shāng Hán Lùn* prescriptions and discussed them here: After first presenting the original text, he then gives the formula's ingredients, quantity, and cooking method, following up with a poem that summarizes all of the above in a way that is easy to memorize. Lastly, he gives some commentary on the formula to explain it further (some of the commentary was added by his grandson).

8. *Yī Xué Cóng Zhòng Lù* 醫學從眾錄 (*A Record of Medicine by Others*): ca. 1819 in eight scrolls. In this book, Chén describes commonly seen diseases of internal medicine and gynecology, and miscellaneous diseases. In each case he describes the pathology, treatment principle, diagnosis, and prescription. He uses eight contemporary scholars' explanations and finishes with Zhāng Zhòngjǐng's explanation. The idea is that the explanations progress from the shallow to the deep. The eight scholars he quotes are Xuē Lìzhāi 薛立齋, Wáng Jīntán 王金壇, Zhào Yǎngkuí 趙養葵, Zhāng Jǐngyuè 張景岳, Zhāng Shíwán 張石頑, Lǐ Shízhēn 李時珍, Lǐ Shìcái 李士材 and Yù Jiāyán 喻嘉言.

9. *Jīn Guì Yào Lüè Qiǎn Zhù* 金匱要略淺注 (*Shallow Commentary on the Jīn Guì Yào Lüè*): ca. 1820 in 10 scrolls. Chén used small print to insert his commentary into the original text, making the Golden Cabinet original text easy to grasp.

10. *Shāng Hán Yī Jué Chuàn Jiě* 傷寒醫訣串解 (*Shāng Hán Medical Method Linked and Explained*): ca. 1821 in six scrolls. In this book, Chén followed the *Shāng Hán Lùn* model and dedicated one scroll to each of the six spheres. In this book Chén crystallized his lifelong research in the classics: He uses the model of root, manifestation, and view from the center, as well as the theory of the channels and network vessels (*jīng luò* 經絡), to explain different difficulties in each sphere. He starts with a question and then replies with a thorough analysis and explanations. In the tàiyáng section, for example, he asks: What is a tàiyáng channel pattern? What is a tàiyáng organ pattern? Why are the promotion of sweating and disinhibiting water the two great methods of treating tàiyáng? This book is a must for anyone studying the *Shāng Hán Lùn*.

11. *Jīn Guì Fāng Gē Kuò* 金匱方歌括 (*Prescriptions from the Golden Cabinet with Poems*): ca. 1830 in six scrolls. Chén compiled 166 prescriptions from the *Jīn Guì Yào Lüè*, in each case inserting first the original text then including a poem to explain the prescription, and lastly a commentary.

12. *Shāng Hán Zhēn Fāng Gē Kuò* 傷寒真方歌括 (*True Prescriptions from the Shāng Hán with Poems*): ca. 1841 in six scrolls. Chén collected ninety-six prescriptions from the *Shāng Hán Lùn*. After presenting a few quotes from the original text, he explains the meaning of the six spheres, pattern differentiation, and treatment methods and then discusses the clinical value of this information in the application of the formulas. In this book he does not follow the *Shāng Hán* sequence when discussing the prescriptions, but instead categorizes the prescriptions according to their nature. Aside from the difference in contents, this is one of the structural differences between this book and the *Cháng Shā Fāng Gē Kuò*.

13. *Nǚ Kē Yào Zhǐ* 女科要旨 (*Essence of Gynecology*): ca. 1841 in four scrolls. The first scroll discusses regulating the menses and fertility. Scroll two discusses gestation, scroll three labor and delivery, and scroll four miscellaneous diseases and external injuries. Chén brings knowledge from the Golden Cabinet and other noted scholars such as Cháo Yuánfāng 巢元方, Chén Zìmíng 陳自明, and Zhū Dānxī 朱丹溪, to thoroughly explain diseases and their remedies.

14. *Yī Xué Shí Zài Yì* 醫學實在易 (*The Study of Medicine is Indeed Easy*): ca. 1844 in eight scrolls. This book synthesizes the different aspects of medicine, from theory to clinical applications. The first scroll contains: "Easy to Know the Viscera and Bowels," "Easy to Know the Channels and Network Vessels," "Easy to Know the Four Diagnostic Methods," and "Easy to Know Qì Transformation." In this format, he summarizes the basic theories of medicine. Scrolls two through four discuss different patterns: external, internal, cold, heat, repletion and vacuity. Each disease is followed by a poem. Scrolls five through seven discuss different formulas and their explanations by different scholars. Scroll eight is an addendum with additional formulas and their modifications.

15. *Shí Yào Shén Shū Zhù Jiě* 十藥神書注解 (*Notes and Explanations on the Divine Book of Ten Herbs*): ca. 1856 in one scroll. Chén's commentary on a book by Gé Kějiǔ 葛可久 (1305-1353 AD), discussing his treatment of tuberculosis. Chén adds in his own clinical experience and critique.

16. *Líng Sù Jié Yào Qiǎn Zhù* 靈素節要淺注 (*Shallow Commentary on Essential Segments of the Líng Shū and Sù Wèn*): ca. 1865 in twelve scrolls. In his last book Chén performs a deep analysis and commentary on segments of the *Líng Shū* and *Sù Wèn*. Oftentimes he uses Zhāng Zhìcōng's commentary in addition to his own developments and explorations of the ancient texts. The book is divided into eleven categories, where different texts with similar contents are pulled together. The categories are: *Dào* of life, Reflections on the Viscera, Channels, Qì Transformation, seeing, hearing, asking, treatment, life and death, pulse diagnosis, and disease mechanism.

Jīn Guì Fāng Gē Kuò 金匱方歌括 (*Prescriptions from the Golden Cabinet with Poems*)

The *Jīn Guì Yào Lüè* 金匱要略 (*Essentials from the Golden Cabinet*) is one of Chinese medicine's most important classics. It was originally written as part of the *Shāng Hán Zábìng Lùn* 傷寒雜病論 (*Treatise on Cold Damage and the Various Diseases*) around 210 AD by Zhāng Zhòngjǐng. As a result of troubling times and frequent warfare, the book was lost for a short period and resurfaced in the hands of the scholar Wáng Shūhé around 270 AD. Wáng rearranged the *Shāng Hán* section of the book into the *Shāng Hán Lùn* or "Treatise on Cold Damage" as we know it today. However, the miscellaneous or Zábìng 雜病 section was missing. It first resurfaced in history during the Táng dynasty in a book named *Wài Tái Mì Yào* 外台秘要 (*Classified Documents of Foreign Official*) by Wáng Táo 王燾 from around 752 AD. It was not until the beginning of the Northern *Sòng* dynasty that Wáng Zhū 王洙, a scholar of the Hànlín 翰林 imperial academy, found among the old books a copy of the *Jīn Guì Yù Hán Yào Lüè Fāng* 金匱玉函要略方. This book was an abridged version of the original *Shāng Hán Zábìng Lùn* in three scrolls. The first scroll covered cold injuries, the second scroll miscellaneous diseases, and the third prescriptions and gynecology. In the eleventh century, the government asked Lín Yì 林億 and other scholars to edit the text and remove the first scroll, which was already published by Wáng Shūhé as *Shāng Hán Lùn*. Only the latter two scrolls about gynecology and miscellaneous diseases were kept in the book. In addition, the editorial team was charged with the task of taking the prescriptions from the end of the book and dividing them up among their corresponding diseases. The new book was to be divided into three scrolls and additional formulas by Zhāng Zhòngjǐng, with other relevant prescriptions from later scholars to be added at the end of the text. This book was named *Treatise on Jīn Guì Yào Lüè Prescriptions*, later referred to most often simply as the *Jīn Guì Yào Lüè*. In this title, *Jīn Guì* refers to a golden cabinet where precious artifacts are kept, while *Yào Lüè* means bare essentials or a summary.

Chén Xiūyuán recognized that the *Jīn Guì Yào Lüè* was known by name by most doctors but its contents were hardly understood. Its text is hard to read and the meaning hidden. Chén explains, "what everyone knows I must not elaborate on … .the title of the book "summary outline" already explains that the text is missing and that mastering the missing parts is the task at hand." Chén furthermore explained that the six-sphere theory in the *Shāng Hán Lùn* is the fundamental theory for the *Jīn Guì* as well. The six spheres do not merely describe cold injuries but rather apply to all diseases. He went further to say that if one wants to learn the *Jīn Guì* he must first know the *Shāng Hán* and the six spheres.

In the *Jīn Guì Fāng Gē Kuò*, Chén continues and deepens his previous work published as *Jīn Guì Yào Lüè Qiǎn Zhù*. Whereas he mainly followed the two Zhāngs from the *Táng* period in his *Shāng Hán Lùn* commentary, in his *Jīn Guì* commentary he uses other scholars and commentaries as a guideline, ultimately utilizing his own enlightened understanding of the ancient text. In this book Chén uses the original text and his own tantalizing poetry and commentary to bring the essence of the *Jīn Guì* prescriptions to the surface. His son Yuánxī continued his father's wishes and provided additional commentary, shedding further light onto the ancient text.

Chén Xiūyuán, a lifelong advocate of the classics and a motivator for following Chinese medicine generations, is one of my scholarly heroes. With a view to the horizon we should follow in his footsteps. This translation of the *Jīn Guì Fāng Gē Kuò* is the first step in this direction.

On this White Dew day in the year Gēng Yín 庚寅 (2010)
In Connecticut, USA
Yaron Seidman
孟亞倫

卷一
Volume One

痙濕暍病方
Jìng Shī Yē Bìng Fāng

Formulas for Tetany, Dampness, and Heat Stroke Diseases

栝蔞桂枝湯
Guā Lóu Guì Zhī Tāng

Trichosanthes and Cinnamon Twig Decoction

治太陽病，其症備，身體強，幾幾然，脈反沉遲，此為痙病。此湯主之。

A treatment for tàiyáng disease with all the symptoms [typical of tàiyáng conditions], rigidity of the body so that it is stretched like a bird about to fly off, but a pulse that is contrary [to our expectations] deep and slow. This means tetany disease. This decoction rules this [condition].

栝蔞根 桂枝 生薑（切）芍藥（各三兩）甘草（二兩，炙）大棗（十二枚，擘）

guā lóu gēn	栝蔞根		9g
guì zhī	桂枝		9g
shēng jiāng	生薑	cut	9g
sháo yào	芍藥		9g
gān cǎo	甘草	honey-fried	6g
dà zǎo	大棗	split	12 pcs

（一）上六味，㕮咀。以水九升，微火煮取三升。（二）溫分三服，微汗。（三）汗不出，食頃，啜熱粥發。

(1) Pound[1] the above six ingredients and boil in 1,800ml of water over a small flame to obtain 600ml.
(2) Take warm, divided into three doses, and induce slight sweating.
(3) If the sweat does not come out, after the amount of time it takes to eat a meal, make the patient sip hot gruel to induce [sweating].

Song 歌曰：

太陽症備脈反沉遲，
身體幾幾欲痙時；
三兩蔞根薑桂芍，
二甘十二棗枚宜。

For conditions with complete tàiyáng symptoms **but** a pulse that is deep and slow,
With the body stretched like a bird about to fly, when the tetany is about to erupt,
Nine grams of *guā lóu gēn, shēng jiāng, guì zhī,* and *sháo yào,*
Six grams of *gān cǎo,* and twelve pieces of *dà zǎo* is the appropriate [treatment].

Commentary by [Chén] Yuánxī[2] 元犀按:

（一）痙是血虛筋燥為病，言濕者，是推其未成痙之前，濕氣挾風，而鬱成內熱也。（二）本條云：太陽症太陽症備，脈反沉遲者，此沉遲乃血虛所致，非臟寒症也。（三）故以桂枝湯和營衛以祛風；加栝蔞根則清氣分之熱，而大潤太陽既耗之液。（四）則經氣流通，風邪自解，濕氣自行，筋不燥而痙愈矣。

(1) Tetany is a disease caused by blood vacuity and dryness in the sinews. When [the text] speaks of dampness, this investigates the stage before the condition has formed tetany, when damp qì that is complicated by wind results in oppression and hence forms internal heat.
(2) When the present paragraph mentions "all the symptoms [typical of tàiyáng conditions] are complete but a pulse that is contrary [to our expectations,] deep and slow," this depth and slowness is due to blood vacuity and is not a symptom of cold in the viscera.
(3) Therefore we use *Guì Zhī Tāng* to harmonize construction and defense to dispel wind. Adding *guā lóu gēn* then clears heat from the qì aspect. [This formula] then

1. *Fǔ jǔ* 㕮咀 translated here as "pound" literally means "chew."

2. Chén Yuánxī was the author's eldest surviving son and the leading figure in arranging and compiling the texts and commentaries of his father and grandfather.

greatly moistens the fluids that have already been consumed in tàiyáng.
(4) As a result, the qì in the channels flows freely, wind evil resolves on its own, damp qì moves on its own, and the sinews are no longer dried out. Thus the tetany is cured!

Additional Commentary 又按:

（一）方中薑、桂合甘、棗，為辛甘化陽。芍藥合甘、棗，為苦甘化陰，陰陽和則得微汗而邪解矣。（二）啜粥則又資陽明之穀氣以勝邪，更深一層立法。(三）但項背幾　幾，脈浮數者，為風淫於外而內之津液未傷，故加葛根以宣外。（四）脈沉遲者，為風淫於外而內之津液已傷，故加栝蔞根以滋內，以栝蔞根苦寒潤燥之功大也。（五）內經云:肺移熱於腎，傳為柔痓。龐安常謂：此方栝蔞根不主項強幾幾，其意以肺熱不令移于腎也。此解亦超。

(1) The *shēng jiāng* and *guì zhī* in the formula combine with *gān cǎo* and *dà zǎo* in acridity and sweetness to transform yáng. *Sháo yào* combines with *gān cǎo* and *dà zǎo* in bitterness and sweetness to transform yīn. The harmony of yīn and yáng then achieves mild sweating and the evil is resolved!
(2) Sipping gruel further enriches grain qì in yángmíng and thereby [aids in] overcoming the evil. On yet one level deeper down, it establishes the method [of treating such conditions].
(3) Nevertheless, if the neck and back are stretched like a bird about to fly but the pulse is floating and rapid, this means that wind excess is on the outside but the fluids on the inside have not yet been damaged. Therefore add *gé gēn* to diffuse the outside.
(4) If the pulse is deep and slow, this means that wind excess is on the outside but the fluids on the inside have already been damaged. Therefore add *guā lóu gēn* to enrich the inside. The effect of using the bitter cold of *guā lóu gēn* to moisten dryness is great.
(5) The *Huáng Dì Nèi Jīng*[3] said: "When the lung transmits heat to the kidney, it spreads to form soft tetany." Páng Ānshí[4] often said: "The *guā lóu gēn* in this formula does not rule the rigidity and stretching of the neck, but its significance lies in the fact that it prevents lung heat from spreading to the kidney. This solution also transcends [this symptom].

3. *Huáng Dì Nèi Jīng* 黃帝內經 refers to the *Hàn* dynasty medical classic that we translate as "Inner Classic of the Yellow Emperor," arguably the single most important text in the history of Chinese medicine.

4. Páng Ānshí was a *Sòng* period physician who specialized in the treatment of Cold Damage disorders. He is most famous for being the author of the *Shāng Hán Zǒng Bìng Lùn* 傷寒總病論 and having invented an alternative formula for *Kǔ Shēn Tāng* 苦參湯.

葛根湯

Gé Gēn Tāng

Pueraria Decoction

歌見長沙方歌括。

For the song, see the *Cháng Shā Fāng Gē Kuò*.[5]

治太陽病，無汗而小便反少，氣上衝胸，口噤不得語，欲作剛痓。此湯主之。

A treatment for tàiyáng disease with no sweating but with urination that is contrary [to our expectations] scant, with qì surging up into the chest, and clenched mouth with inability to speak. This is a condition in which hard tetany is about to erupt. This decoction rules this [condition].

葛根（四兩）麻黃（三兩，去節）桂枝（二兩，去皮）芍藥（二兩）生薑（三兩，切）大棗（十二枚，掰）甘草（二兩，炙）

gé gēn	葛根		12g
má huáng	麻黃	knots removed	9g
guì zhī	桂枝	bark removed	6g
sháo yào	芍藥		6g
shēng jiāng	生薑	cut	9g
dà zǎo	大棗	split	12 pcs
gān cǎo	甘草	honey-fried	6g

(一)上七味，㕮咀，以水一斗，先煮麻黃葛根，減二升。(二)去沫，內諸藥，煮取三升，去滓。(三)溫服一升，覆取微似汗，不須啜粥。(四)余如桂枝湯法將息及禁忌。

(1) Pound the seven ingredients above. First simmer the *má huáng* and *gé gēn* in

5. This refers to *Formulas with Songs from Cháng Shā*, a companion book of commentary and songs on the *Shāng Hán Lùn* formulas written by Chén Xiūyuán.

2,000ml of water until reduced by 400ml.
(2) Remove the foam, add all the other medicinals, and simmer until reduced to 600ml. Remove the dregs.
(3) Take 200ml per dose heated, and cover [the patient] with a blanket to induce mild sweating. You do not have to [make the patient] sip gruel.
(4) For further instructions, follow the methods applying to *Guì Zhī Tāng* as far as rest and contraindications are concerned.

Commentary by [Chén] Yuánxī 元犀按:

（一）無汗例用麻黄湯，然惡其太峻。（二）故於桂枝湯加麻黄以發汗。（三）君葛根以清經絡之熱，是發表中寓養陰之章也。（四）又此方與前方皆是太陽中兼陽明之藥，以陽明主宗筋也。

(1) In cases without sweating, you would ordinarily use *Má Huáng Tāng*. Nevertheless, I detest its excessive fierceness.
(2) Therefore [the formula here] uses *Guì Zhī Tāng* with the addition of *má huáng* to effuse sweat.
(3) By clearing the heat from the channels and network vessels, the sovereign *gé gēn* has the significance of also nourishing yīn in the midst of effusing the exterior.
(4) Moreover, both this formula and the previous one are medicines for tàiyáng in combination with yángmíng, because yángmíng rules the ancestral sinews.

大承氣湯

Dà Chéng Qì Tāng

Major Qì Coordinating Decoction

歌見長沙方歌括 。

For the song, see the *Cháng Shā Fāng Gē Kuò*.

治痙病，胸滿，口噤，臥不著席，腳攣急，必齘齒 。可與此湯 。

A treatment for tetany conditions with fullness in the chest and clenched mouth, not touching the mat when lying on the back, hypertonicity in the legs, and invariably also grinding of the teeth. You can give this formula [to treat such conditions].

大黃（ 四兩，酒洗 ）厚朴（ 半斤，炙，去皮 ）枳實（ 五枚，炙 ）芒硝（ 三合 ）

dà huáng	大黃	washed in liquor	12g
hòu pò	厚朴	honey-fried and skin removed	24g
zhǐ shí	枳實	honey-fried	5 pcs
máng xiāo	芒硝		60ml

（ 一 ）上四味，以水一斗，先煮枳朴，取五升 。（ 二 ）去滓，內大黃，煮取二升 。（ 三 ）去滓，內芒硝，更上微火一二沸 。（ 四 ）分溫再服 。（ 五 ）得下止服 。

(1) Of the four ingredients above, simmer *zhǐ shí* and *hòu pò* in 2,000ml of water until reduced to 1,000ml.
(2) Remove the dregs, add the *dà huáng*, and simmer until reduced to 400ml.
(3) Remove the dregs, add the *máng xiāo*, and again place it on a small flame to boil once or twice.
(4) Divide and take heated in two doses.
(5) As soon as precipitation [i.e. defecation] is achieved, stop taking it.

Commentary by [Chén] Yuánxī 元犀按:

（一）胸滿、口噤、腳攣急、齘齒等證，皆熱甚灼筋，筋急而甚之象。（二）以此湯急下而救陰。（三）齘牙藥不能進，以此湯從鼻中灌之。（四）三承氣湯歌解，見于長沙方歌括。

(1) The various symptoms like fullness in the chest, clenched mouth, hypertonicity in the legs, grinding teeth, etc. all are manifestations of severe heat scorching the sinews, so that the sinews become tense, aggravating the symptoms even further.
(2) Use this formula to precipitate urgently and rescue yīn.
(3) If [the patient] is unable to consume the medicine because of the grinding of the teeth, pour the decoction in through the nose.
(4) For songs with explanations on the three [modifications of] *Chéng Qì Tāng*, see the *Cháng Shā Fāng Gē Kuò.*

麻黄加朮湯

Má Huáng Jiā Zhú Tāng

Ephedra Decoction With White Atractylodes Added

治濕家身煩疼。發其汗為宜，慎不可以火攻之。宜此湯主之。

A treatment for patients suffering from dampness with generalized vexation and aching. It is suitable to promote sweating, but beware: You must not use fire to attack [the dampness]. It is suitable to use this decoction to rule [such conditions].

麻黄（三兩，去節）桂枝（二兩）甘草（一兩，炙）白朮（四兩）杏仁（七十個，去皮尖）

má huáng	麻黄	nodes removed	9g
guì zhī	桂枝		6g
gān cǎo	甘草	honey-fried	3g
bái zhú	白朮		12g
xìng rén	杏仁	skin and tops removed	70 pits

（一）上五味，以水九升，先煮麻黄，減二升。（二）去上沫，內諸藥，煮取二升半，去滓。（三）溫服八合。覆取微汗。

(1) Of the five ingredients above, first boil the *má huáng* in 1,800ml of water until reduced by 400ml.
(2) Remove the foam on the surface, toss in the various [other] medicinals, and simmer until reduced to 500ml. Remove the dregs.
(3) Take 160ml [as one dose], heated. Cover [the patient] to cause mild sweating.

Song 歌曰：

煩疼濕氣裹寒中，
發汗為宜忌火攻；

莫訝麻黄湯走表，
朮加四兩裡相融。

For vexation and aching from damp qì being wrapped inside cold,
Promoting sweating is suitable, but fire attack is contraindicated.
Never be surprised that *Má Huáng Tāng* runs to the exterior,
While the addition of twelve grams of *bái zhú* causes melting in the interior.

Commentary by [Chén] Yuánxī 元犀按:

（一）身煩疼者，寒濕之邪著於膚表也。（二）膚表實，故無汗；無汗，則邪無從出矣。（三）方用麻黄湯發膚表之汗，以散表寒。（四）又恐大汗傷陰，寒去而濕反不去，加白朮補土生液，而助除濕氣，此發汗中寓緩汗之法也。（五）又白朮補脾驅濕之功甚大，且能助脾之轉輸而利水。（六）觀仲祖用朮各方可知。（七）今人炒燥，炒黑，上蒸，水漂等制，皆失經旨。

(1) The generalized vexation and aching is [due to] the evils of cold and dampness adhering to the skin on the exterior.
(2) Because the skin on the exterior is replete, there is no sweating. As the result of no sweating, the evil has no place from whence to emerge!
(3) The formula uses *Má Huáng Tāng* to promote sweating from the skin on the exterior, thereby dispersing exterior cold.
(4) Now because we fear that great sweating will damage yīn, so that the cold is removed but the dampness is on the contrary not removed, we add *bái zhú* to supplement earth and engender the fluids, thereby assisting in eliminating damp qì. This is the method of promoting sweating by means of moderate sweating.
(5) Moreover, the effect of *bái zhú* in supplementing the spleen and driving out dampness is great indeed and can also assist in the spleen's activity of moving and disinhibiting water.
(6) You can know this from the fact that Ancestor Zhòng[6] uses *bái zhú* in every formula.
(7) Nowadays, people process it by dry-roasting it, roasting it until blackened, steaming it, or letting it float on water. All of these [methods of preparation] have lost the intention of the classic.

6. This refers to the author of the *Jīn Guì Yào Lüè* 金匱要略, namely Zhāng Zhòngjǐng 張仲景.

麻黃杏仁薏苡甘草湯

Má Huáng Xìng Rén Yì Yǐ Gān Cǎo Tāng

Ephedra, Apricot Kernel, Coix, and Licorice Decoction

治病者一身盡疼，發熱日晡所劇者，此名風濕。此病傷於汗出當風，或久傷取冷所致也。

A treatment for patients who suffer from aching all over their entire body and heat effusion that is aggravated during dusk. This condition is called wind-damp. In this disease, the damage has come from exposure to wind while sweating or from long-term damage from catching cold.

麻黃（半兩）杏仁（十個，去皮尖）薏苡（半兩）甘草（一兩，炙）

má huáng	麻黃		1.5g
xìng rén	杏仁	skin and tops removed	10 pits
yì yǐ rén	薏苡仁		1.5g
gān cǎo	甘草	honey-fried	3g

（一）上銼麻豆大，每服四錢匕。（二）水一盞半，煎八分，去滓。（三）溫服，有微汗，避風。

(1) Grate the above ingredients to the size of *má dòu.*[7] For each dose take four *qián*-spoons full.[8]
(2) Boil it down in one-and-a-half cups of water to eight tenths and remove the dregs.
(3) Take it heated. There will be mild sweating. Avoid [exposure to] wind.

---

7. "Hemp beans", aka hemp seeds.

8. 方寸匕者，作匕正方一寸，抄散取不落為度。錢匕者，以大錢上全抄之。
"For a square-inch spoon, make a spoon that is exactly the size of a one-*cùn* square and measure out a full spoon of powder without dropping any. For a *qián*-spoon, take everything that can fit on top of a large *qián* coin." *Bèi Jí Qiān Jīn Yào Fāng* 備急千金要方, vol. 1.

Song 歌曰:

風濕身疼日晡時,
濕無去來, 風有休息,
與上節濕家分別在此。
當風汗出, 當風取冷, 久傷取冷病之基;
薏麻半兩十枚杏,
炙草扶中予其勝濕之權一兩宜。

In wind-damp, there is generalized aching around dusk.
While dampness has neither past nor future, wind has periods of rest.
By this sign, we differentiate it from the cases of dampness described above.
Exposure to wind, **i.e. exposure to wind when sweating**, and catching cold, **i.e. long term damage from cold**, are the foundations of disease.
Two grams each of *yì yǐ rén* and *má huáng*, ten pits of *xìng rén*.
Of honey-fried *gān cǎo* to support the center, three grams is appropriate **to give the power to overcome dampness.**

Comparison 參:

(一) 以上二方, 為濕家立法也。(二) 又有風濕之證, 其痛輕掣不可屈伸, 非如濕家之痛, 重著不能轉側。(三) 且濕家發熱, 旦暮不殊, 風濕發熱, 日晡增甚。(四) 晡, 申時也。陽明旺於申酉戌, 土惡濕。(五) 今為風濕所干, 當其旺時, 邪正相搏, 則反劇也。(六) 濕無去來, 風有休作, 故名風濕。(七) 然言風, 寒亦在其中。現原文云: 汗出當風, 或久傷取冷, 意可知矣。(八) 蓋痙病非風不成, 濕痹無寒不作。(九) 方中麻黄散寒; 意苡除濕; 杏仁利氣, 助麻黄驅寒之力; 甘草補中, 予意苡勝濕之權。(十) 制方之糟密如此。

(1) The two formulas above establish treatment methods for patients suffering from dampness.
(2) Furthermore, the sign of wind-damp is that the pain is mild with tugging and inability to bend and stretch. This is not like the pain in patients suffering from dampness, which is severe and accompanied by inability to turn to the side.
(3) Moreover, in patients suffering from dampness the heat effusion is no different at dawn and at dusk, but in wind-damp conditions, the heat effusion is greatly increased during dusk.
(4) Dusk is the time of *shēn* [i.e., 3-5 pm]. Yángmíng is exuberant during the times of

shēn, *yǒu* [5-7 pm], and *xū* [7-9 pm]. Earth is averse to dampness.
(5) The condition at hand is due to an invasion of wind-damp, and during the time of its exuberance, evil and right struggle with each other. As a result it is more fierce then.
(6) Because dampness has neither past nor future but wind has times of resting and of activity, this condition is called wind-damp.
(7) Nevertheless, when [the text] speaks of wind, there is also cold in it. Consider this quote from the original source: "Exposure to wind when sweating or long-term damage from catching cold." You can know its meaning from this.
(8) Now tetany disease is invariably generated by wind, and damp impediment can never arise without cold.
(9) In the formula, ***má huáng*** dissipates cold; ***yì yǐ rén*** eliminates dampness; ***xìng rén*** disinhibits qì and aids ***má huáng*** in its action of driving out cold; ***gān cǎo*** supplements the center and gives ***yì yǐ rén*** the power to overcome dampness.
(10) The precision of the prepared formula is like this.

防己黄芪湯

Fáng Jĭ Huáng Qí Tāng

Fáng Jĭ and Astragalus Decoction

治風濕，脈浮，身重，汗出惡風者主之。

A treatment for conditions of wind-damp with a floating pulse, generalized heaviness, sweating, and aversion to wind. [This formula] rules these [symptoms].

防己（一兩）甘草（半兩，炙）白朮（七錢半）黄芪[9]（一兩一分，一本用一兩）

fáng jĭ	防己		3g
gān căo	甘草	honey-fried	1.5g
bái zhú	白朮		2.25g
huáng qí	黄芪		3.75g

（一）上銼麻豆大，每服五錢匕，生薑四片，大棗一枚，水盞半，煎八分。去滓，溫服。（二）喘者加麻黄半兩。胃中不和者加芍藥三分。氣上衝加桂枝三分。下有陳寒者加細辛三分。（三）服後當如虫行皮中，從腰下如冰。後坐被上，又以一被繞腰下，溫令微汗，差。

(1) Grate the above ingredients to the size of *má dòu*. For each dose, take five *qián*-spoons full. With four pieces of *shēng jiāng* and one piece of *dà zăo*, simmer [each dose] in half a cup of water [until reduced] to eight tenths. Remove the dregs and take heated. (2) For panting, add one-and-a-half grams of *má huáng*. For disharmony in the stomach, add two-and-a-quarter grams of *sháo yào*. For upsurging qì, add two-and-a-quarter grams of *guì zhī*. For stale cold in the lower body, add two-and-a-quarter grams of *xì xīn*. (3) After taking [this decoction], it will feel like bugs moving inside the skin and from the waist down like ice. Then have [the patient] sit on top of a blanket and wrap them in another blanket below the waist. Keep them warm to induce mild sweating. [This means] recovery.

9. Another edition uses 3g.

Song 歌曰:

身重脈浮汗，
上節無汗，故用麻黃發之；
此節汗出，止用防己驅之。
惡風，七錢半朮五錢甘草通，
己芪一兩磨分服，
每服五錢匕。
四片生薑一棗充 。

Generalized heaviness, a floating pulse, and sweating,
[as opposed to] the previous section, where there was no sweating and the formula therefore used *má huáng* to promote it.
In the present section, there is sweating, so to stop it you use *fáng jǐ* to drive it out.
For the aversion to wind, two-and-a-quarter grams of *bái zhú* and one-and-a-half grams of *gān cǎo* promote free flow.
With three grams each of *fáng jǐ* and *huáng qí*, grind the ingredients up and take in separate doses,
each dose consisting of five *qián*-spoons full.
Four pieces of *shēng jiāng* and one *dà zǎo* complete [the formula].

Attached Song for Modifications 附加減歌:

喘者再入五錢麻 。
胃不和兮芍藥加 。
三分分字去聲讀，
七錢五分今不差，
寒取細辛，氣衝桂，
俱照三分效可夸 。
服後如蟲行皮里，
腰下如冰，取被遮，
遮繞腰溫得微汗 。
伊岐秘法闡長沙 。

For panting, further add one-and-a-half grams of *má huáng*;
For disharmony of the stomach, *sháo yào* is added,
Three *fèn* [two-and-a-quarter grams], whereby the character "fen" (分) is read in fourth tone.[10]

10. The significance of this line is unclear and might be related to a change in pronunciation over time. In modern usage, the character 分, when read in first tone, means "to divide" and from there by extension "fraction," as well as serving as a unit of measurement. In fourth tone, it means "component" or "portion."

With six grams, nothing is missing today.
For cold, take *xì xīn*; for qì surges, *guì zhī*.
All of these are efficacious when added [in the amount of] two-and-a-quarter grams.
After taking [this decoction], it is as if there were bugs moving inside the skin
And like ice below the waist. Take a blanket to cover [the patient].
Also cover [the patient] around the waist and warm them up until there is mild sweating.
This is Yī and Qí's secret method that they have clarified for the man from Cháng Shā.[11]

Comparison 合參:

（一）上方治實邪無汗，即桂枝、麻黄二湯例也。（二）虛汗自出，故不用麻黄以散之。只用防己以驅之。（三）服後如蟲行，及腰下如冰云云，皆濕氣下行之征也。（四）然非芪、朮、甘草，焉能使衛陽復振而驅濕下行哉?

(1) The previous formula treats repletion evil without sweating, which the two decoctions *Guì Zhī Tāng* and *Má Huáng Tāng* illustrate.
(2) [In the present formula], we see spontaneous discharge of vacuity sweat. So we do not use *má huáng* to dissipate it. Only use *fáng jǐ* to drive it out.
(3) After taking [the formula], the feelings of bugs moving and of ice below the waist both are evidence of damp qì moving downward.
(4) Nevertheless, without *huáng qí, bái zhú,* and *gān cǎo,* how could you cause defensive yáng to be revitalized to drive dampness out from the lower body?

Commentary by [Chén] Yuánxī 元犀按:

（一）張隱庵本草經注云：防己生于漢中者，破之紋如車輻稿，莖藤空通，主通氣行水，以防己土之藥，故有防己之名。（二）金匱治水、治痰諸方，蓋取氣運于上，而水能就下也。（三）李東垣渭防己乃下焦血分之藥，上焦氣分者禁用等論。（四）張隱庵歷歷指駁，使東垣聞之，當亦俯首無詞。（五）噫!不讀神農本經而妄為臆說，甘為伊岐之罪人，復何責焉？（六）防己功用，余先君注有神農本草經，議論甚詳，毋庸再贅。

11. This is a reference to Zhāng Zhòngjǐng, who was from Cháng Shā.

(1) Zhāng Yǐn'ān[12] said in his notes to the "*Shén Nóng Běn Cǎo Jīng*"[13]: "*Fáng jǐ* grows in the River Hàn, and when you break it, its lines are like the spokes in wheels. The stalks and canes are hollow and continuous. It's key action is to promote the free flow of qì and to move water. Because *fáng jǐ* is a medicinal of earth, therefore it has the name *fáng jǐ* ["guarding yīn earth"]."
(2) All the formulas in the *Jīn Guì Yào Lüè* that treat water or phlegm use the method of transporting qì to the upper body, as a result of which water can then be precipitated.
(3) Lǐ Dōngyuán[14] refered to *fáng jǐ* as a medicinal of the lower burner and blood aspect and has discussed such ideas as that it is contraindicated for the upper burner and the qì aspect.
(4) Zhāng Yǐn'ān has distinctly pointed out this contradiction. He caused the words of Lǐ Dōngyuán to be heard but could only bow his head and remain speechless.
(5) Alas! To rashly make assumptions and speak without having read the *Shén Nóng Běn Cǎo Jīng*, you will of your own accord become someone who transgresses against Yī and Qí.[15] How could they then get blamed for that?
(6) On the effect of *fáng jǐ*, my deceased father commented on the *Shén Nóng Běn Cǎo Jīng* where he debated it in minute detail. There is no need for redundancy here.

12. Zhāng Yǐn'ān 張隱庵 was a *Qīng* dynasty author famous for his commentaries on the *Sù Wèn*, *Líng Shū*, and *Shén Nóng Běn Cǎo Jīng*.

13. The Divine Farmer's Classic of Materia Medica (神農本草經, *Hàn* dynasty).

14. Lǐ Dōngyuán 李東垣, also known as Lǐ Gǎo 李杲, was one of the "Four Masters of the *Jīn-Yuán* period 金元四大家, the author of the *Pí Wèi Lùn* 脾胃論 (*Treatise on the Spleen and Stomach*), and the founder of the Supplementing-Earth School (*bǔ tǔ pài* 補土派). His dates are 1180-1251.

15. Yī 伊 is a reference to a mythological figure named 伊尹, who served King Tāng 湯 of the *Shāng* dynasty as his chef, giving him advice on government while serving him the medicinal soups he had prepared. Qí is a reference to Qí Bó 岐伯, the personal physician and advisor of the Yellow Emperor who is most famous for the dialogues with the Yellow Emperor recorded in the *Huáng Dì Nèi Jīng*.

桂枝附子湯

Guì Zhī Fù Zǐ Tāng

Cinnamon Twig and Aconite Decoction

傷寒八九日，風濕相搏，身体疼煩，不能自轉側，不嘔不渴，脈浮虛而濇者，桂枝附子湯主之。若大便堅，小便自利者，去桂加白朮湯主之。

On the eighth or ninth day of cold damage, wind and dampness struggle with each other, [manifesting in] generalized pain and vexation, inability to turn to the side on your own, no retching or thirst, and a floating, vacuous and rough pulse. *Guì Zhī Fù Zǐ Tāng* rules this [condition]. If the stools are hard but urination is naturally disinhibited, take out the *guì zhī* but add *bái zhú* in the decoction to rule it.

桂枝（四兩，去皮）生薑（三兩，切）附子（三枚，炮去皮，破八片）甘草（二兩，炙）大棗（十二枚，擗）

guì zhī	桂枝	bark removed	12g
shēng jiāng	生薑	cut	9g
fù zǐ	附子	blast-fried, skin removed, broken into 8 pieces	3 pcs
gān cǎo	甘草	honey-fried	6g
dà zǎo	大棗	split	12 pcs

上五味，以水六升，煮取二升，去滓，分溫三服。

Simmer the five ingredients above in 1,200ml of water until reduced to 400ml. Remove the dregs and take heated in three doses.

白朮附子湯

Bái Zhú Fù Zǐ Tāng

White Atractylodes and Aconite Decoction

白朮（二兩）附子（一枚半，炮去皮）甘草（一兩，炙）生薑（一兩半，切）大棗（六枚，掰）

bái zhú	白朮		6g
fù zǐ	附子	blast-fried, skin removed	1.5 pcs
gān cǎo	甘草	honey-fried	3g
shēng jiāng	生薑	cut	4.5g
dà zǎo	大棗	split	6 pcs

（一）上五味，以水三升，煮取一升，去滓，分溫三服。（二）一服覺身痹，半日許再服。（三）三服都盡，其人如冒狀，勿怪。即是朮附并走皮中，逐水氣，未得除故耳。

(1) Simmer the five ingredients above in 600ml of water until reduced to 200ml. Remove the dregs, divide and take heated in three doses.
(2) After one dose, [the patient] will feel generalized impediment. After half a day, take a second dose.
(3) When the three doses are all used up, the person might have the appearance of veiling. Do not consider this strange. The reason for this is that *bái zhú* and *fù zǐ* together are running into the skin to expel water qì but have not been able to eliminate it yet.

甘草附子湯

Gān Cǎo Fù Zǐ Tāng

Peony, Licorice, and Aconite Decoction

甘草（二兩，炙）白朮（二兩）附子（二枚，炮去皮）桂枝（四兩，去皮）

gān cǎo	甘草	honey-fried	6g
bái zhú	白朮		6g
fù zǐ	附子	blast-fried, skin removed	2 pcs
guì zhī	桂枝	bark removed	12g

（一）上四味，以水六升，煮取三升，去滓。溫服一升，日三服。（二）初服得微汗則解。（三）能食汗出复煩者，服五合。恐一升多者，服六、七合為妙。

(1) Simmer the four ingredients above in 1,200ml of water until reduced to 600ml. Remove the dregs and take 200ml [per dose] heated, three doses per day.
(2) If the initial dose promotes mild sweating, [the condition] is resolving.
(3) If [the patient] is able to eat but the vexation returns with sweating, take [an additional] 100ml. If you fear that 200ml is too much, it is excellent to take 120ml or 140ml.

以上三方歌解，證治俱見長沙方歌括。

For songs, explanations, evidence, and treatments concerning the three formulas above, see the *Cháng Shā Fāng Gē Kuò*.

白虎人參湯

Bái Hǔ Rén Shēn Tāng

White Tiger and Ginseng Decoction

歌見長沙方歌括。

For the song, see the *Cháng Shā Fāng Gē Kuò.*

太陽中熱者，暍是也。汗出惡寒，身熱而渴者主之。

When tàiyáng is struck by heat, this is heat stroke. For sweating with aversion to cold, generalized heat, and thirst, [this formula] rules.

知母（六兩）石膏（一斤，碎）甘草（二兩）粳米（六合）人參（三兩）

zhī mǔ	知母		18g
shí gāo	石膏	smashed	48g
gān cǎo	甘草		6g
jīng mǐ	粳米		120ml
rén shēn	人參		9g

上五味，以水一斗煮，米熟，汤成。去滓，温服一升，日三服。

Simmer the five ingredients above in 2,000ml of water until the rice [*jīng mǐ*] is cooked and the decoction is done. Remove the dregs and take 200ml heated, three doses per day.

Commentary by [Chén] Yuánxī 元犀按:

（一）白虎，西方神名也。其令為秋，其政清肅。（二）涼風至，白露降，則溽暑潛消。（三）以此湯有徹暑熱之功，行清肅之政，故以白虎名之。

(1) White tiger is the name of the spirit of the Western direction. Its command is autumn, its governance is to clear and depurate.
(2) When the cool winds arrive and white dew[16] falls, the sweltering heat of summer disappears.
(3) Because this decoction has the effect of piercing through the heat of summer and performs the governmental task of clearing and depurating, therefore it is named after White Tiger.

16. White dew can refer literally to the frost that is beginning to appear on cool autumn mornings, or to the season of "White Dew," which begins around September 8th in the Western calendar.

栝蒂散

Guā Dì Sǎn

Melon Stalk Powder

治太陽中暍，身熱疼重而脈微弱 。此以夏月傷冷水，水行皮中所致也 。此湯主之 。

A treatment for heat stroke in tàiyáng, with generalized heat, aching and heaviness, and a faint weak pulse. This [condition] is caused by damage from cold water during the summer months, when the water has moved into the skin. This decoction rules this [condition].

栝蒂 二七個

guā dì	栝蒂	27 pcs

上銼，以水一升煮取五合，去滓，溫服 。

Grate the above [ingredient] and simmer in 200ml of water until reduced to 100ml. Remove the dregs and take heated.

Song 歌曰：

暍病，陰陽認要真，
熱疼身重得其因 。
暑為濕戀名陰暑，
二七甜栝蒂可珍 。

In the disease of heat stroke, yīn and yáng each want to be perfected.
Heat is where the aching and heaviness of the body find their cause.
Summerheat is complicated by dampness, hence the name "yīn summerheat."
Twenty-seven stalks of sweet *guā dì* can be a treasure.

Commentary by [Chén] Yuánxī 元犀按:

此物能去水氣，水去則暑無所依而自愈矣。

This substance is able to remove water qì. When water qì is removed, summerheat has nothing to lean against and is cured by itself.

Quotation by Yóu Zàijīng[17] 尤在涇云:

（一）暑雖陽邪，而氣恆與濕相合，陽求陰之義也。（二）暑因濕入，而暑反居濕之中，陰包陽之象也。

(1) Even though summerheat is a yáng evil, its qì commonly combines with dampness. The significance of this is that yáng is seeking yīn.
(2) Summerheat enters because of dampness, and then summerheat contrary [to our expectations] resides within dampness. This is a manifestation of yīn enveloping yáng.

Another quote 又云:

（一）暑之中人也，陰虛而多火者，暑即寓于火之中，為汗出而煩渴。（二）陽虛而多濕者，暑即伏于濕之內，為身熱而疼重。（三）故暑病恒以濕為病，而治濕即所以治暑。（四）栝蒂苦寒，能吐能下，去身、面、四肢水氣，水去而暑解。（五）此治中暑兼濕者之法也。

(1) When summerheat strikes a person, if the person suffers from yīn vacuity and a profusion of fire, this means that summerheat is residing in the midst of fire, which manifests as sweating followed by vexation and thirst.
(2) If the person suffers from yáng vacuity and a profusion of dampness, the summerheat will become latent inside the dampness, which means generalized heat, aching, and heaviness.
(3) Therefore such conditions of summerheat are eternally complicated by dampness, and treating dampness is the way in which we treat [this kind of] summerheat.
(4) *Guā dì* is bitter and cold and is able to induce vomiting and precipitation. It removes water qì from the body, face, and four extremities, and once the water is removed, the summerheat is also resolved.
(5) This is the method for treating heat stroke complicated by dampness.

17. A famous physician from the *Qīng* dynasty (?~1749) who composed several commentaries on the *Shāng Hán Lùn* and *Jīn Guì Yào Lüè*.

百合狐惑陰陽毒方
Bǎi Hé Hú Huò Yīn Yáng Dú Fāng

Formulas for Hundred-Union,[18] Fox-Creeper,[19] and Yīn-Yáng-Toxin Diseases

Summarizing Song 總歌:

Quote on Hundred-Union disease in particular 百合尤云:

百脈朝於肺，以肺為主。
病從百脈成，
起居冒昧各難名。
藥投，吐利如神附，
頭痛參觀溺更明。
以溺時頭痛為辨，
蓋百脈之所重，
在少陰、太陽，以太陽統六經之氣，
其經上循巅頂，
下通水道，氣化不行，
乃下溺而上頭痛。
少陰為生水之源，
開合澀乃溺而淅然。

The hundred vessels are presided over by the lung and the lung is their ruler.
Diseases arise from the hundred vessels,
But their periods of activity and rest are rash and obscure so that it is difficult to name each.
[As the result of] having given medicine,
[the patient responds with] vomiting and disinhibition as if there were spirits involved.
You can observe the headaches, and the urination is an even more obvious [sign].
Headache at the time of urination

18. The World Health Organization (WHO) glosses this as an "ancient term for neurosis characterized by mental strain, listlessness, sleeplessness, anorexia, pseudo heat and pseudo cold, bitterness in the mouth, yellow urine and rapid pulse." *WHO International Standard Terminologies on Traditional Medicine in the Western Pacific Region*, (World Health Organization, 2006), p.168.

19. "A disease characterized by erosion of the mouth, throat and genitalia, red eyes and black canthi, resembling Behcet's syndrome." Ibid., p. 184.

can be used to differentiate the importance of the hundred vessels:
Whether shàoyīn or tàiyáng, since tàiyáng controls the qì in the six channels,
And its channel runs upward to encircle the top of the head,
And frees the flow in the waterways in the lower body, if qì transformation does not move,
There will be urinating below and headache above.
Shàoyīn is the source of generating water,
And when opening and closing are inhibited, urination is followed by shivering.

百合知母湯

Bǎi Hé Zhī Mǔ Tāng

Lily Bulb and Anemarrhena Decoction

百合病發汗後者，此方主之。

After patients with Hundred-Union disease have been [erroneously treated with] sweating, this formula rules.

百合（十枚）知母（三兩）

bǎi hé	百合	10 pcs
zhī mǔ	知母	9g

（一）上先以水洗百合，漬一宿，當白沫出。（二）去其水，別以泉水二升煎取一升，去滓。（三）別以泉水二升煎知母，取一升。（四）後合煎取一升五合，分溫再服。

(1) Of the above ingredients, first wash the *bǎi hé* in water and soak overnight until white foam appears.
(2) Drain the water and again simmer in 400ml of spring water until reduced to 200ml. Remove the dregs.
(3) Separately, simmer the *zhī mǔ* in 400ml of spring water until reduced to 200ml.
(4) Afterwards combine [the two fluids] and simmer together until reduced to 300ml. Divide and take heated in two doses.

百合知母湯

Song 歌曰:

病非應汗汗傷陰，
知母當遵三兩箴；
漬去沫涎七枚百合，
別煎泉水是金針。
諸方煎法俱同。

In this disease, you should not treat by sweating because sweating damages yīn.
Regarding the *zhī mǔ*, you must obey the warning about the nine grams.
Soak seven **pieces** of *bǎi hé* and remove the foam.
Separately simmering them in spring water, this is the Golden Needle.
The method of simmering is identical in all the various formulas.

Commentary by [Chén] Yuánxī 元犀按:

（一）百脈俱朝於肺，百脈俱病，病形错雜，不能悉治，只於肺治之。（二）肺主氣，氣之為病，非實而不順，即虛而不足。（三）百合能治邪氣之實，而補正氣之虛；知母入肺金，益其水源，下通膀胱，使天水之氣合，而所傷之陰，轉則其邪從小便出矣。（四）若誤汗傷陰者，汗為陰液，陰液傷，故以此湯維其陽，維陽即所以救陰也。

(1) The hundred vessels are all presided over by the lung, and when the hundred vessels are all diseased, the disease forms are misleading and complex. You cannot treat them all thoroughly. You can only treat them by means of the lung.
(2) The lung rules qì and the way in which qì manifests in disease is either through repletion and lack of smooth flow, or in vacuity and insufficiency.
(3) *Bǎi hé*[20] is able to treat repletion of evil qì and supplements vacuity of right qì. *Zhī mǔ* enters lung metal, boosts its water source, frees the bladder in the lower body, causes the qì of heaven's water to unite and transforms the yīn that has been damaged so that the evil is discharged through the urine.
(4) If erroneous sweating has damaged yīn, since sweat is a yīn fluid and yīn fluids are therefore damaged, this decoction ties together yáng and by tying together yáng rescues yīn.

20. The Chinese characters for *bǎi hé*, the name of the key medicinal in this formula, literally translated mean "hundred unions."

Quotation by Wáng Jìnsān[21] 王晉三云：

（一）本文云百脈一宗，明言病歸於肺，君以百合，甘涼清肺，即此可療此疾。（二）再佐以各經清解絡熱之藥，治其病所從來。（三）當用先後煮法，使不悖于手足經各行之理。（四）若誤汗傷太陽者，溺時頭痛，以知母救肺之陰，使膀胱水府知有母氣，救肺即所以救膀胱，是陽病救陰之法也。

(1) When this text said that the hundred vessels share a common ancestor, it means that disease returns to the lung. *Bǎi hé* is the sovereign [of this formula], which with sweetness and coolness clears the lung. Hence the disease can be cured in this way.
(2) Moreover, assisted by a medicinal that clears and resolves heat in the network vessels in each channel, [the formula] treats the location whence the disease originated.
(3) You must use the method of simmering [the ingredients separately] first and then [add them] together, so that you do not go against the principle of the flow in each of the hand and foot channels.
(4) If erroneous sweating has damaged tàiyáng, there will be headache at the time of urination. Use *zhī mǔ* to rescue the yīn of the lung and let the palace of water, namely the bladder, know that qì of its mother is available. By rescuing the lung you hence rescue the bladder. This is the method of [treating] yáng disease by rescuing yīn.

21. An honored government official and physician who lived from 1698-1761.

百合滑石代赭石湯

Bǎi Hé Huá Shí Dài Zhě Shí Tāng

Lily Bulb, Talcum, and Hematite Decoction

百合病下之後者，此湯主之 。

After patients with Hundred-Union disease have been [erroneously treated with] precipitation, this decoction rules.

百合（ 七枚，擘 ）滑石（ 三兩，碎，綿裹 ）代赭石（ 如彈丸大一枚，碎，綿裹 ）

bǎi hé	百合	split	7 pcs
huá shí	滑石	smashed, wrapped in gauze	9g
dài zhě shí	代赭石	smashed, wrapped in gauze	1 pc the size of a pellet

（ 一 ）上先煎百合如前法 。（ 二 ）別以泉水二升煎滑石 、代赭石，取一升 。（ 三 ）去滓後合和重煎，取一升五合 。（ 四 ）分溫服五合 。

(1) Of the ingredients above, first simmer the *bǎi hé* as in the previous formula.
(2) Separately simmer the *huá shí* and *dài zhě shí* in 400ml of spring water until reduced to 200ml.
(3) After removing the dregs, combine [with the *bǎi hé* liquid] and simmer again until reduced to 300ml.
(4) Divide and take heated, 100ml per dose.

Song 歌曰:

不應議下下之差，
既下還當竭舊邪;
百合七枚赭彈大，
滑須三兩效堪夸 。

You should not consider precipitation [as treatment in Hundred-Union disease]. The shortcoming of precipitation is that the precipitation will further drive the old evil to its utmost.
Seven pieces of *bǎi hé*, a pellet-sized piece of *dài zhě shí*,
Nine grams of *huá shí*, and the effect can be praised.

Commentary by [Chén] Yuánxī 元犀按:

（一）誤下者，其熱必陷，熱陷必傷下焦之陰。（二）故以百合清補肺金，引動水源。（三）以代赭石鎮離火，而不使其上騰。（四）以滑石導熱氣，而能通水府。（五）則所陷之邪從小便而出，自無灼陰之患矣。（六）此即見陽救法也。

(1) Erroneous precipitation invariably causes the heat to be trapped, and the entrapment of heat invariably damages yīn in the lower burner.
(2) Therefore, [this formula] uses *bǎi hé* to clear and supplement lung metal and to guide and move the water source.
(3) It uses *dài zhě shí* to settle heart fire and prevent it from soaring upward.
(4) It uses *huá shí* to draw out the heat and is thereby able to free the palace of water.
(5) As a result, the entrapped evil is discharged through the urine and there is no more worry about burning yīn.
(6) This is the method of rescuing by making yáng visible.

Commentary by Wáng Jìnsān 王晉三云:

（一）誤下傷少陰者，溺時淅然，以滑石上通肺，下通太陽之陽。（二）恐滑石通府利竅，仍蹈出汗之弊，乃復代赭石重鎮心經之氣，使無汗泄之虞。（三）是陰病救陽之法也。

(1) In conditions where erroneous precipitation has damaged shàoyīn, we see shivering at the time of urinating. Use *huá shí* to free the flow in the lung in the upper body and free the yáng in tàiyáng in the lower body.
(2) Fearing that *huá shí* frees the bowels and disinhibits the orifices, we skip the disadvantage of expelling sweat and [instead] use the heaviness of *dài zhě shí* to settle the qì in the heart channel, allowing us to avoid any apprehension about sweating and discharging [i.e. inducing diarrhea].
(3) This is the method of [treating] yīn disease by rescuing yáng.

百合雞子黃湯

Bǎi Hé Jī Zǐ Huáng Tāng

Lily Bulb and Egg Yolk Decoction

百合病吐之後者，此方主之。

After patients with Hundred-Union disease have been [erroneously treated with] vomiting, this formula rules.

百合（七枚）雞子黃（一枚）

bǎi hé	百合	7 pcs
egg yolk	雞子黃	1 pc

（一）上先煎百合如前法，取一斗。（二）去滓，內雞子黃攪勻，煎五分，溫服。

(1) Of the above ingredients, first simmer the *bǎi hé* in the same manner as above until reduced to 2,000ml.
(2) Remove the dregs, add the egg yolk, and stir until evenly mixed. Simmer until reduced by five tenths and take heated.

Song 歌曰:

不應議吐吐傷中，
中者陰之守也。
必伏陰精上奉功；
內經云：陰精上奉，其人壽。
百合七枚洗去沫，
雞黃後入攪渾融。

You should not consider vomiting because vomiting damages the center.
The center is the guardian of yīn.
It invariably subdues the effect of yīn essence supporting the upper body.

The *Nèi Jīng* said, "when yīn essence supports the upper body, the person is long lived."
Take seven pieces of *bǎi hé*, rinse them, and remove the foam.
Afterwards, add *jī huáng* and mix well until blended.

Commentary by [Chén] Yuánxī 元犀按:

(一）吐後傷中者，病在陰也。（二）陰傷，故用雞子黄養心胃之陰，百合滋肺氣，下潤其燥。（三）胃為肺母，胃安則肺氣和而令行。（四）此亦用陰和陽，無犯攻陽之戒。

(1) In conditions where the center has been damaged after vomiting, the disease is in yīn.
(2) Because yīn is damaged, use egg yolk to nourish the yīn in the heart and stomach and *bǎi hé* to enrich lung qì and moisten the dryness in the lower body.
(3) The stomach is the mother of the lung, and when the stomach is quieted, lung qì is harmonious and commands movement.
(4) This [formula] also uses yīn to harmonize yáng. Do not violate the prohibition against attacking yáng.

Quotation by Wáng Jìnsān 王晉三云:

(一）誤吐傷陽明者，以雞子黄救厥陰之陰。（二）以安胃氣，救厥陰，即所以奠陽明，救肺之母氣。（三）是亦陽病救陰之法也。

(1) For conditions where erroneous [induction of] vomiting has damaged yángmíng, use egg yolk to rescue yīn in juéyīn.
(2) By quieting stomach qì and rescuing juéyīn, you will thereby settle yángmíng and rescue the qì of the lung's mother.
(3) This is also a method for treating yáng disease by rescuing yīn.

百合地黃湯

Bǎi Hé Dì Huáng Tāng

Lily Bulb and Rehmannia Decoction

百合病，不經吐，下，發汗，病形如初者，此湯主之 。

In Hundred-Union disease, if the patient has not been treated by inducing vomiting, precipitation, or sweating, and the outside form of the disease is the same as at the onset, this decoction rules it.

百合（ 七枚 ）生地黃汁（ 一升 ）

bǎi hé	百合	7 pcs
shēng dì huáng zhī	生地黃汁	200ml of juice

（ 一 ）上洗 。（ 二 ）煎百合如前法，取一升，去滓 。（ 三 ）內地黃汁，煎取一升五合，溫分再服 。（ 四 ）中病勿更服 。大便當如漆 。

(1) Wash the above ingredients.
(2) Simmer the *bǎi hé* as in the method described in the previous formulas until reduced to 200ml, and remove the dregs.
(3) Add the *dì huáng* juice and simmer until reduced to 300ml. Take heated, divided into two doses.
(4) When the disease is struck, do not give any further doses. The stool should look like lacquer.

Song 歌曰:

不經汗下吐諸傷，
形但如初守太陽；
遷延日久，始終在太陽經不變者；
地汁一升百合七，
陰柔最是化陽剛 。

In patients who have not suffered the various damages from sweating, precipitation, and vomiting,
Where the form of the disease is still just as at the onset abiding in tàiyáng,
From beginning to end always in the tàiyáng channel without any change,
200ml of *dì huáng* juice and seven pieces of *bǎi hé*
Are the most effective at using yīn softness to transform yáng hardness.

Commentary by [Chén] Yuánxī 元犀按:

（一）病久不經吐、下、發汗，病形如初者，是鬱久生熱，耗傷氣血矣。（二）主之百合地黃湯者，以百合苦寒清氣分之熱，地黃汁甘潤泄血分之熱，皆取陰柔之品以化陽剛。（三）為泄熱救陰法也。（四）中病者，熱邪下泄，由大便而出矣，故曰如漆色。

(1) In cases where the disease has been chronic but the patient has not undergone induced vomiting, precipitation, and sweating, where the form of the disease is still like at the onset, chronic depression has engendered heat and consumed qì and blood.
(2) The reason *Bǎi Hé Dì Huáng Tāng* rules this condition is that the bitterness and coldness of *bǎi hé* clears heat from the qì aspect, while the sweetness of *dì huáng* juice moistens and discharges heat from the blood aspect. In both cases, we take a substance of yīn softness to transform yáng hardness.
(3) This is the method of rescuing yīn by discharging heat.
(4) "When the disease is struck" means that the heat evil has been discharged and is emerging in the stool. Therefore the stool is said to be the color of lacquer.

百合洗方

Bǎi Hé Xǐ Fāng

Formula for Bǎi Hé Rinse

百合病一月不解，變成渴者，此方主之。

When Hundred-Union disease has persisted for one month without being resolved, and has transformed into thirst, this formula rules.

百合（一升）

bǎi hé 百合 200ml

（一）上以百合（一升），以水一斗，漬之一宿。（二）以洗身。（三）洗已，食煮餅，勿以鹽豉也。

(1) For the above, soak 200ml of *bǎi hé* in 2,000ml of water over one night.
(2) Use it to wash the patient.
(3) After washing, eat boiled wheat cakes, but do not eat salted fermented beans.

Song 歌曰：

月周不解渴因成，
邪熱流連肺不清；
百合一升水一斗，
洗身食餅不和羹。
勿以鹽豉。

If not resolved in an entire month and thirst is engendered because of it,
Evil heat has spread into the lung instead of clearing.
With 200ml of *bǎi hé* in 2,000ml of water,
Wash the body and then eat wheat cakes but not in combination with broth.
Do not eat salted fermented beans.

Comparison 合參:

（一）皮毛為肺之合，洗其外，亦所以通其內也。（二）又食煮餅者，假麥氣，穀氣以輸津。（三）勿以鹽豉者，恐鹽味耗水以增渴也。

(1) The skin and hair are the connection to the lung. Washing the outside [of the body] also thereby frees the flow on the inside.
(2) Moreover, eating boiled wheat cakes means availing ourselves of the qì of wheat,[22] hence using grain qì to transport the liquids.
(3) The prohibition against consuming salted fermented beans is related to the fear that the salty flavor wears on water and thereby increases the thirst.

22. According to traditional Chinese dietetics, wheat is more moistening than other grains and thus assists the fluids.

栝蔞牡蠣散

Guā Lóu Mǔ Lì Sǎn

Trichosanthes and Oyster Shell Powder

百合病渴不差者，此散主之。

For patients with Hundred-Union disease when the thirst does not improve, this powder rules.

栝蔞根 牡蠣（熬，等分）

guā lóu gēn	栝蔞根	
mǔ lì	牡蠣	boiled in water

上為細末，飲服方寸匕，日三服。

Process equal amounts of the above ingredients into a fine powder and take one gram in fluid, three doses a day.

Song 歌曰：

洗而仍渴屬浮陽，
牡蠣蔞根並等量；
研末飲調方寸匕，
寒兼咸苦苦寒，咸寒效逾常。

Unabated thirst after being washed is associated with floating yáng.
Mǔ lì and *guā lóu gēn* in equal amounts,
Grind into a powder and drink in doses of one gram.
The effect of cold with salty and bitter [medicinals] **i.e., bitter cold and salty cold** is extraordinary.

Commentary by [Chén] Yuánxī 元犀按:

（一）洗後而渴不差，是內之陰氣未復。（二）陰氣未復，由於陽氣之亢。（三）故用牡蠣以潛其 陽，栝蔞根以生其津，津生陽降，而渴愈矣。

(1) Conditions where the thirst does not improve after the patient has been washed [with the decoction above] are ones in which yīn qì on the inside has not recovered yet.
(2) The reason that yīn qì has not recovered is the hyperactivity of yáng qì.
(3) Therefore, the formula uses *mǔ lì* to subdue yáng and *guā lóu gēn* to engender liquid. When liquid is engendered and yáng brought down, the thirst is cured!

百合滑石散

Bǎi Hé Huá Shí Sǎn

Lily Bulb and Talcum Powder

百合病，變發熱者，此散主之。

For patients with Hundred-Union disease that has transformed into heat effusion, this powder rules.

百合（一兩，炙）滑石（三兩）

bǎi hé	百合	honey-fried	3g
huá shí	滑石		9g

（一）上為散，飲服方寸匕，日三服。（二）當微利者止服，熱則除。

(1) Process the above ingredients into a powder and take one gram in fluid, three doses per day.
(2) When there is mild diarrhea, stop taking [any additional] doses. This heat is being eliminated.

Song 歌曰:

前此寒無熱亦無，
首章言如寒無寒，如熱無熱。
變成發熱熱堪虞。
清疏滑石宜三兩，
百合烘篩一兩需。

[In the conditions described] before this [formula], there was no cold and also no heat.
As the initial paragraph of the chapter [in the *Jīn Guì Yào Lüè*] describes, "a condition that looks like cold but without cold, that looks like heat but without heat."
When this condition transforms into heat effusion, the heat is very troublesome.

Of clearing and coursing *huá shí*, nine grams are suitable;
Of toasted and sifted *bǎi hé*, three grams are needed.

Commentary by [Chén] Yuánxī 元犀按:

（一）百合病原無偏熱之證。（二）變發熱者，內熱充滿，淫於肌膚，非如熱之比。（三）主以百合滑石散者，百合清金瀉火降逆氣，從高源以導之；滑石退表里之熱，利小便，二味合為散者。（四）取散以散之之義，散調絡脈于周身，引內外之熱氣，悉從小便出矣。

(1) Hundred-Union disease originally does not manifest with the sign of tendency towards heat.
(2) When the condition transforms into heat effusion, [it means that] heat is overfull on the inside so that it oozes into the skin. This does not resemble a [regular] heat condition.
(3) The reason *Bǎi Hé Huá Shí Sǎn* rules this condition is that *bǎi hé* clears metal, drains fire, and downbears counterflow qì, thereby leading it down from its high source, while *huá shí* abates the heat in the interior and exterior and disinhibits urine. The two ingredients are combined into a powder.
(4) Choosing the form of a powder (散) has the significance of dispersing (散) it. Powder harmonizes the network vessels all over the body, drawing out the heat qì from the inside and outside so that it is completely discharged through the urine.

甘草瀉心湯

Gān Cǎo Xiè Xīn Tāng

Licorice Heart-Draining Decoction

（一）治狐惑病，狀如傷寒，默默欲眠，目不得閉，臥起不安。（二）蝕於喉為惑，蝕於陰為狐。（三）不欲飲食，惡聞食臭，其面目乍赤、乍黑、乍白。（四）蝕於上部則聲嗄，宜此湯。（五）蝕於下部則咽干，宜苦參湯洗之。（六）蝕於肛者，雄黃熏之。

(1) A treatment for Fox-Creeper Disease, which manifests in an appearance like in cold damage, deep silence and desire to sleep, inability to close the eyes, and restlessness whether at rest or active.
(2) When the erosion is found in the throat, it is called "creeper." When the erosion is found in the area of the genitals and anus, it is called "fox."
(3) The patient has no desire to drink or eat and is averse to the smell of food. The face and eyes are sometimes red, sometimes black, sometimes white.
(4) When the erosion is located in the upper body, it results in a hoarse voice. [In that case,] this decoction is suitable.
(5) When the erosion is located in the lower body, it results in a dry throat. [In that case,] it is suitable to wash it with *Kǔ Shēn Tāng*.
(6) When the erosion is in the anus, fumigate it with *xióng huáng*.

甘草（四兩，炙）黃芩 乾薑 人參（各三兩）半夏（半升）黃連（一兩）大棗（十二枚）

gān cǎo	甘草	honey-fried	12g
huáng qín	黃芩		9g
gān jiāng	乾薑		9g
rén shēn	人參		9g
bàn xià	半夏		100ml
huáng lián	黃連		3g
dà zǎo	大棗		12 pcs

上七味，以水一斗，煮取六升，去滓，再煎取三升，溫服一升，日三服。

Simmer the seven ingredients above in 2,000ml of water until reduced to 1,200ml. Remove the dregs and simmer again until reduced to 600ml. Take 200ml heated, three doses a day.

Song 歌曰:

傷寒論中甘草瀉心湯，
卻妙增參三兩匡。
彼治痞成下利甚，
此醫狐惑探源方。

Gān Cǎo Xiè Xīn Tāng from the *Shāng Hán Lùn*
Is indeed ingenious when assisted by the addition of nine grams of *rén shēn*.
Elsewhere treating glomus[23] that is giving rise to severe diarrhea,
This is a formula that explores the source of treating fox creeper.

Commentary by [Chén] Yuánxī 元犀按:

（一）蟲有情識，故能亂有情識之心臟而生疑惑矣。（二）蟲為血化之物，故仍歸於主血之心。（三）方且類聚群分，若有妖妄，憑借而然，其實不外本身之血氣以為祟耳。（四）此方補虛而化濕熱，雜以辛苦之味，名曰瀉心，意深哉!

(1) Worms have affection and knowledge. Therefore they are able to cause upheaval in the heart viscus, which has affection and knowledge, and engender doubt and confusion.
(2) Worms are a substance of blood transformation and therefore return to the heart, which rules the blood.
(3) Now things are divided into different categories according to their nature, and if there is something monstrous and weird [in the patient's condition], it is so by relying on [the affinity between worms and the heart]. The true reality of what is causing the calamity is nothing that is external to the blood and qì of the patient's body.
(4) This formula supplements vacuity and transforms damp heat, by mingling acrid and bitter flavors. It is called "draining the heart." Its meaning is deep indeed!

23. Wiseman glosses this as "A localized subjective feeling of fullness and blockage." *A Practical Dictionary of Chinese Medicine*, second edition by Nigel Wiseman and Feng Ye (Paradigm Publications, 1999), p. 242.

苦參湯

Kŭ Shēn Tāng

Flavescent Sophora Decoction

Editorial comment:

龐安時傷寒總病論用苦參半斤，槐白皮、狼牙根各四兩，煎，熏洗之。

The *Shāng Hán Zǒng Bìng Lùn*[24] by Páng Ānshí, uses twenty-four grams of ***kŭ shēn*** and twelve grams each of ***huái bái pí*** and ***láng yá gēn***, simmered and used as a steam wash.

苦參（一升）

kŭ shēn	苦參	200ml

以水一斗，煎取七升，去滓，熏洗，日三。

Simmer in 2,000ml of water until reduced to 1,400ml. Remove the dregs and [apply to the genitals as] a steam wash, three times a day.

24. *Treatise on All the Diseases of Cold Damage*. The author of the text, Páng Ānshí was a famous physician and author from the Northern *Sòng* period, who lived ca. 1042 ~ 1099.

雄黃熏法
Xióng Huáng Xūn Fǎ
Method of Fumigation with *Xióng Huáng*

雄黃一味為末，筒瓦二枚合之，燒，向肛熏之 。

Process the single ingredient *xióng huáng* into a powder, place two barrel tiles together and burn [the *xióng huáng*] in it. Fumigate [the patient by directing the smoke] towards the anus.

Song 歌曰:

苦參湯是洗前陰，
下蝕從下而衝於上咽乾熱最深；
更有雄黃熏法在，
肛門蟲蝕亦良箴 。
蝕在肛者發癢，俗呼臟頭風。

Kǔ Shēn Tāng is used to wash the genitals
For erosion in the lower body, **surging upward from below,** with dry throat and deepest heat,
You can also apply the method of fumigating with *xióng huáng*.
This is also an excellent warning to the worms eroding the entrance to the anus.
Erosion at the anus causing itching is commonly called "wind at the head of the viscera."

Commentary by [Chén] Yuánxī 元犀按:

（一）蝕於喉為惑，蝕於陰為狐。（二）狐惑病乃感風木濕熱之氣而生，寒極而化也。（三）苦參苦寒，氣清屬陽，洗之以通陽道；雄黃苦寒，氣濁屬陰，熏之以通濁道。（四）但雄黃稟純陽之色，取其陽能勝陰之義也。（五）熏洗二法，按陰陽分配前後二陰，此又別其陰中之陰陽也。（六）二味俱苦寒而燥者，苦以瀉火，寒以退熱，燥以除濕，濕熱退而蟲不生矣。

(1) Erosion in the throat is called "creeper." Erosion in the area of the genitals and anus is called fox.

雄黃熏法

(2) Fox-Creeper disease is engendered by contracting the qì of damp-heat in wind-wood and transformed by extremes of cold.
(3) *Kǔ shēn* is bitter and cold. Its qì is clear and belongs to yáng. Wash with it to free the path of yáng. *Xióng huáng* is bitter and cold. Its qì is turbid and belongs to yīn. Fumigate with it to free the turbid path.
(4) Nevertheless, *xióng huáng* is endowed with the color of pure yáng.[25] The significance is that it takes its yáng and is thereby able to overcome yīn.
(5) To apply the two methods of fumigation and washing, assign them in accordance with yīn and yáng to the anterior and posterior yīn [i.e. the genitals and anus respectively]. This is again how you differentiate between yīn in yīn and yáng in yīn.
(6) The two ingredients are both bitter and cold as well as drying. Bitterness is used to drain fire, cold is used to abate heat, and dryness is used to eliminate dampness. When damp-heat abates, worms are no longer generated!

25. The Chinese name literally means "male yellow."

赤小豆當歸散

Chì Xiǎo Dòu Dāng Guī Sǎn

Rice Bean and Chinese Angelica Powder

治脈數，無熱，微煩，默默但欲臥，汗出，初得之三四日，目赤如鳩眼，七八日，目四眦黑。若能食者，膿已成也。此方主之。並治先便後血。

A treatment for [conditions manifesting with] rapid pulse, absence of heat, mild vexation, deep silence and only wanting to lie down, sweating, and during the first three or four days of contracting this disease red eyes like those of a turtle dove, but after seven or eight days blackness in the four corners of the eyes. If the patient is able to eat, pus has already formed. This formula rules [this condition]. It also treats bleeding after elimination [of feces and urine].

赤小豆（三升，浸令芽出，曝乾）當歸（十分）

chì xiǎo dòu	赤小豆	soaked until sprouted and then dried in the sun	600ml
dāng guī	當歸		7.5g

上二味，杵為散，漿水服方寸匕，日三服。

Process the two ingredients above by pestling them into a powder. Take one gram in fermented grain-water,[26] three doses a day.

Song 歌曰：

眼眦赤黑變多般，
小豆生芽曝令干；
豆取三升歸十分，
杵調漿水日三餐。

For redness or blackness in the corners of the eyes changing in so many ways,
Chì xiǎo dòu that has sprouted and been dried in the sun.

26. This refers to an ancient beverage, produced by adding cool water to the hot cooked grains and letting the mixture stand and ferment for 5-7 days until it is slightly sour with white foam on the top but not spoiled.

Take 600ml of beans and seven-and-a-half grams of *dāng guī*,
Pestle and mix with fermented grain-water, three meals a day.

Commentary by [Chén] Yuánxī 元犀按:

（一）此治濕熱侵陰之病，大抵濕變為熱，則偏重於熱。（二）少陰主君火，厥陰主風木，中見少陽相火。（三）病入少陰，故見微煩，默默但欲臥等證；病人厥陰，故目赤現出火色，目眦黑，現出火極似水之色。（四）主以赤豆去濕，清熱解毒，治少陰之病；當歸導熱養血，治厥陰之病；下以漿水，以和胃氣。（五）胃氣與少陰和，則為火土合德;胃氣與厥陰和，則為土木無忤。微乎！微乎！

(1) This [formula] is a treatment for conditions where damp-heat has invaded yīn. In most cases, dampness transforms into heat, resulting in an abnormal predominance on heat.
(2) Shàoyīn rules the sovereign fire, juéyīn rules wind-wood, and in the middle we see the ministerial fire in shàoyáng.
(3) Because the disease has entered shàoyīn, we see signs like mild vexation, and deep silence, and only wanting to lie down. Because the patient is affected in juéyīn, we see redness in the eyes, which is the color of fire emerging, and blackness in the corners of the eyes, which is a manifestation of the color of extreme fire resembling water.
(4) Rule this condition by means of *chì xiǎo dòu* to remove dampness, clear heat, and resolve toxins, to treat the disease in shàoyīn. Use *dāng guī* to draw out heat and nourish blood, to treat the disease in juéyīn. Down the formula with fermented grain-water to harmonize stomach qì.
(5) When stomach qì is harmonious with shàoyīn, the virtue of fire and earth is combined. If stomach qì is harmonious with juéyīn, earth and wood do not resist each other. Profound indeed! Profound indeed!

Another commentary 又按:

（一）或謂是狐惑病，或謂是陰陽毒病，然二者皆濕熱蘊毒之病。
（二）金匱列於二證交界處，即是承上起下法。

(1) Some call this disease Fox-Creeper Disease, some call it Yīn-Yáng Toxin Disease. Nevertheless, the two terms both refer to a disease of damp-heat brewing toxin.
(2) The way in which the *Jīn Guì Yào Lüè* lines up these two signs in interaction is thus merely a method of continuing with the previous to raise the latter.

升麻鱉甲湯

Shēng Má Biē Jiǎ Tāng

Cimicifuga and Turtle Shell Decoction

治陽毒病，面赤斑斑如錦紋，咽喉痛，吐膿血，五日可治，七日不可治，此湯主之。

A treatment for yáng toxin disease, [which manifests in] a red face with spots all over resembling the lines in brocade, sore throat, and spitting of pus and blood, treatable within five days but untreatable after seven days. This decoction rules it.

升麻（二兩）當歸甘草（各一兩）蜀椒（炒去汗，一兩）鱉甲（手指大一片，炙）雄黃（半兩，研）

shēng má	升麻		6g
dāng guī	當歸		3g
gān cǎo	甘草		3g
shǔ jiāo	蜀椒	stir-fried until the "sweat" is gone	3g
biē jiǎ	鱉甲	honey-fried	1 pc the size of a finger
xióng huáng	雄黃	ground into dust	1.5g

（一）上六味，以水四升，煮取一升，頓服之。（二）老小再服。取汗。（三）陰毒去蜀椒、雄黃。

(1) Simmer the six ingredients above in 1,200ml of water until reduced to 200ml. Take it by drinking it down in one gulp.
(2) For old or young patients, divide into two doses. It will make the patient sweat.
(3) For yīn toxin, remove the *shǔ jiāo* and *xióng huáng*.

升麻鱉甲湯

Song 歌曰：

面赤斑紋咽痛毒為陽，
鱉甲周圍一指量，
半兩雄黃升二兩，
椒歸一兩草同行 。

In [patients with] a face marked by redness, **spots, and lines,** and a sore throat, the toxin is yáng.
An amount of *biē jiǎ* in circumference like a single finger,
One-and-a-half grams of *xióng huáng* and six grams of *shēng má,*
Three grams of *shǔ jiāo* and *dāng guī,* and the same amount of *gān cǎo.*

Commentary by [Chén] Yuánxī 元犀按:

（一）非常災癘之氣，從口鼻而入咽喉，故陰陽二毒皆咽痛也。
（二）陰陽二證，不以寒熱臟腑分之，但以面赤斑紋，吐陳血，其邪著于表者，謂之陽；面目青，身痛如被杖，其邪隱于表中之里者，為陰。

(1) [In this condition], the qì of unusually disastrous pestilence has entered the throat from the mouth and nose. Therefore both yīn toxin and yáng toxin manifest with sore throat.
(2) We do not differentiate the evidence for yīn and yáng by heat or cold or by viscera and bowels, but by the redness in the face with spots and lines and spitting of stale blood, which signify that the evil is attached to the exterior and we therefore call it a yáng condition, or by the green-blue face and eyes and generalized pain as if beaten with a staff, which signify that the evil is hidden in the interior inside the exterior, making it a yīn condition.

升麻鱉甲湯去雄黃蜀椒

Shēng Má Biē Jiǎ Tāng Qù Xióng Huáng Shǔ Jiāo

Cimicifuga and Turtle Shell Decoction Without Realgar and Zanthoxylum

治陰毒病，面目青，身痛如被杖，咽喉痛，五日可治，七日不可治，此湯主之。

A treatment for yīn toxin disease, [which manifests in] a green-blue face and eyes, generalized pain as if the person had been beaten with a staff, and sore throat, treatable within five days but untreatable after seven days. This decoction rules it.

升麻（二兩）當歸甘草（各一兩）鱉甲（手指大一片，炙）

shēng má	升麻		6g
dāng guī	當歸		3g
gān cǎo	甘草		3g
biē jiǎ	鱉甲	honey-fried	1 pc the size of a finger

Song 歌曰：

身疼咽痛面皮青，
陰毒苛邪隸在經，
陰毒以面不赤而青，身不斑紋而痛如被杖別之，
二証俱咽痛，俱五日可治，七日不可治。
即用前方如法服，
四味照前法服。
椒黃務去特丁寧。
蜀椒、雄黃二物，陽毒用之者，以陽從陽，欲其速散也，
陰毒去之者，恐陰邪不可劫，而陰氣反受損也。

Generalized pain, sore throat, and a green-blue skin color in the face
[Are the evidence] that yīn toxin is tormenting and that the evil belongs to the channels.
You differentiate yīn evil by the fact that the face is not red but green-blue and that the body is not marked by spots and lines but suffers pain as if beaten with a staff.
Both [yīn and yáng toxin conditions] share the sign of sore throat
and both can be treated within the first five days but not after seven days.
Promptly use the method described in the previous formula to dose it

升麻鱉甲湯去雄黃蜀椒

And take the four ingredients as in the above method.

It is a particularly serious warning that *shǔ jiāo* and *xióng huáng* must be removed.

The two ingredients *shǔ jiāo* and *xióng huáng* that are used for yáng toxin, use yáng to follow yáng, to dissipate it speedily.

We remove them in patients with yīn toxin becuase of the fear that they will injure yīn qì rather then assault yīn evil.

Quotation by Wáng Jìnsān 王晋三云：

（一）升麻入陽明、太陽二經，升清逐穢，辟百邪，解百毒，統治溫癘陰陽二病。（二）如陽毒為病，面赤斑如錦紋；陰毒為病，面青，身如被杖；咽喉痛，毋論陰陽二毒，皆已入營矣。（三）但升麻僅走二經氣分，故必佐當歸通絡中之血，甘草解絡中之毒，微加鱉甲守護營神，俾椒、黃猛劣之品攻毒透表，不能亂其神明。（四）陰毒去椒、黃者，太陽主內，不能透表，恐反動癘毒也。（五）肘後千金方陽毒無鱉甲者，不欲其守，亦恐留戀癘毒也。

(1) *Shēng má* enters the yángmíng and tàiyáng channels, upbearing the clear and driving out the filthy, repelling the hundred evils, and controlling warm pestilence in both yīn and yáng disease.
(2) If yáng toxin causes the disease, the face is red with spots resembling the lines in brocade. If yīn toxin causes the disease, the face is green-blue and the body feels as if it had been beaten with a staff. The sign of sore throat is present regardless of whether it is related to yīn or to yáng toxin, and in both cases means that the disease has already entered construction.
(3) Nevertheless, *shēng má* only runs into the qì aspect of the two channels. We therefore require the assistance of *dāng guī* to free the flow of blood in the network vessels and that of *gān cǎo* to resolve the toxin in the network vessels, with a small addition of *biē jiǎ* to guard the spirit and construction. As a result, the *shǔ jiāo* and *xióng huáng*, which are products with a fierce strength, attack the toxin and outthrust the exterior but are unable to derange the spirit light.
(4) The reason we remove *shǔ jiāo* and *xióng huáng* in yīn toxin conditions is that tàiyáng rules the inside and is unable to outthrust the exterior, so we fear that it will conversely stir the toxin of pestilence.
(5) The reason the formulas for yáng toxin in the *Zhǒu Hòu Bèi Jí Fāng*[27] and *Bèi Jí Qiān Jīn Yào Fāng*[28] do not include *biē jiǎ* is that they do not desire its guarding [effect] and fear that instead it will make the toxin of pestilence lodge and adhere.

27. *Prescriptions [to Carry] Behind the Elbow* 肘後備急方 (Gě Hóng 葛洪, 281–341).

28. *Essential Prescriptions Worth a Thousand in Gold for Every Emergency* 備急千金要方 (Sūn Sīmiǎo 孙思邈, 7th century).

卷二
Volume Two

瘧病方
Nüè Bìng Fāng

Formulas for Malaria Disease

鱉甲煎丸
Biē Jiǎ Jiān Wán
Turtle Shell Brew Pills

治瘧病以月一日發，當十五日愈。設不瘥，當月盡解。如其不瘥，結為症瘕。名曰瘧母，急治之。宜此丸主之。

A treatment for malaria that erupts on the first day of the [lunar] month, in which case recovery should occur on the fifteenth day.[29] If the patient fails to recover, it should resolve at the very end of the month. If the patient [still] fails to recover, [the malaria] will bind to form concretions and conglomerations. This conditions is called "mother of malaria" and must be treated immediately. It is suitable to treat it with these pills. They rule it.

鱉甲（十二分，炙）烏扇[30]（三分，燒，即射乾）黃芩（三分）柴胡（六分）鼠婦（三分，熬）乾薑 大黃 桂枝 石韋（去毛）厚朴 紫葳[31]（即淩霄）半夏 阿膠 芍藥 牡丹皮 䗪蟲（各五分）葶藶 人參（各一分）瞿麥（二分）蜂窠[32]（四分，炙）赤硝（十二分）蜣螂（六分，熬）桃仁（二分）

biē jiǎ	鱉甲	honey-fried	9g
wū shàn	烏扇	roasted	2.25g

29. The first day of the lunar month is the day of the new moon, and the fifteenth day is the day of the full moon.

30. *Wū shàn* is an alternate name for *shè gān* 射乾 (Rhizome of Belamcanda chinensis).

31. I.e., *líng xiāo* 淩霄 (Flower of Campsis grandiflora).

32. *Fēng wō* is an alternate name for *fēng fáng* 蜂房 (Nest of Vespae nidus).

huáng qín	黃芩		2.25g
chái hú	柴胡		4.5g
shǔ fù	鼠婦	boiled in water	2.25g
gān jiāng	乾薑		2.25g
dà huáng	大黃		2.25g
guì zhī	桂枝		2.25g
shí wéi	石韋	hair removed	2.25g
hòu pò	厚朴		2.25g
zǐ wēi	紫葳		2.25g
bàn xià	半夏		3.75g
ē jiāo	阿膠		2.25g
sháo yào	芍藥		3.75g
mǔ dān pí	牡丹皮		3.75g
zhè chóng	䗪蟲		3.75g
tíng lì	葶藶		0.75g
rén shēn	人參		0.75g
qū mài	瞿麥		1.5g
fēng wō	蜂窠	honey-fried	3g
chì xiāo	赤硝		9g
qiāng láng	蜣螂	boiled in water	4.5g
táo rén	桃仁		1.5g

（一）上二十三味，為末。（二）取煅灶下灰一斗，清酒一斛五升，浸灰，俟酒盡一半。（三）著鱉甲於中，煮令泛爛如膠漆，絞取汁。（四）內諸藥，煎為丸，如梧於大。（五）空心服七丸，日三服。

(1) Process the twenty-three ingredients above into a powder.
(2) Take 2 liters of glowing hot ashes from the bottom of a stove and soak them in 11 liters of clear liquor. Wait until half the liquor has evaporated.
(3) Then add the *biē jiǎ*. Simmer until it has a mushy consistency like glue or lacquer. Squeeze to get the liquid.
(4) Add all the other medicinals, make a brew and then make pills from it, the size of parasol tree seeds.
(5) On an empty stomach take seven pills per dose, three doses a day.

附：千金方用鱉甲十二片，又有海藻三分，大戟一分，無鼠婦、赤硝二味。

Attached note: The *Bèi Jí Qiān Jīn Yào Fāng* uses twelve slices of ***biē jiǎ***, and moreover adds two-and-a-quarter grams of ***hǎi zǎo*** and three-quarters-of-a gram of ***dà jǐ***, but does not include the two ingredients ***shǔ fù*** and ***chì xiāo***.

Song 歌曰:

寒熱虛實相來往，
全憑陰陽為消長。
天氣半月而一更，
人身之氣亦相仿。
否則天人氣再更，
邪行月盡差可想，
瘧病一月不能瘥，
瘧母結成癥瘕象。
金匱急治特垂訓，
鱉甲赤硝十二分，
方中三分請詳言，
薑芩扇婦朴韋問，
葳膠桂黃亦相均，
相均端令各相奮。
君不見十二減半六分數，
柴胡蜣螂表里部，
一分參蘗二瞿麥桃仁，
牡夏芍䗪虫分各五，
方中四分獨蜂窠，
體本經清質水土，
另取灶下一斗灰，
一斛半酒浸另服，
納鱉甲酒內煮如膠，
絞汁煎藥末丸遵古。
空心七丸日服三，
每服七丸，一日三服也。
盧子繇痎瘧疏方云，
漸加一十一丸。
老瘧得此效桴鼓。

Whether cold or heat, vacuity or repletion come and go
Completely depends on the growth and decline of yīn and yáng.

Heaven's qì completes one cycle of change in half a month,[33]
And the qì in the human body is also like this.
If [malaria] is not [cured], the qì of heaven and of the human body starts another cycle.
When evil runs into the very end of the month, recovery is thinkable.
If malaria is not cured in one month,
The mother of malaria will bind and form the appearance of concretions and conglomerations.
In the *Jīn Guì Yào Lüè,* immediate treatment is a teaching especially emphasized.
Biē jiă and *chì xiāo,* nine grams each;
In the formula, medicinals used in two-and-a-quarter gram amounts please speak of with care.
For *gān jiāng, huáng qín, wū shàn, shŭ fù, hòu pò,* and *shí wéi,* ask!
Zĭ wēi, ē jiāo, guì zhī, dà huáng are also in equal proportions.
The equal amounts cause each of them to struggle with the other.
Do you not see, sir, that nine reduced by half **amounts to four and a half grams?**
Chái hú and *qiāng láng* for the exterior and interior parts,
Three-quarters-of-a gram of *rén shēn* and *tíng lì* and one-and-a-half grams of *qū mài* and *táo rén,*
Mŭ dān pí, bàn xià, sháo yào and *zhè chóng,* each in three and three-quarter gram amounts.
In the formula, three grams are only used for *fēng wō.*
The body originally passes through pureness in a substance of water and earth.
In addition, **take** 2,000ml of ashes from the bottom of the stove,
Also take 15,000ml of liquor to soak it in,
Add the *biē jiă* to the liquor and simmer until it resembles glue,
Ring out the liquid, brew the medicine, and form the powder into pills, following the old ways.
On an empty stomach, seven pills, three doses daily,
Each dose seven pills, three doses a day.
Master Lú[34] said in a formula that allows malaria to disperse
To gradually increase [the dosage] to eleven pills.
In old malaria, you obtain instantaneous effects like [the sound from] sticks on a drum.

Quotation by Yóu Zàijīng 尤在涇云:

（一）天氣十五日一更，人之氣亦十五日一更，氣更則邪當解也。（二）否則三十日天人之氣再更，而邪自不能留矣。（三）設更不愈，其邪必假血依痰，結為癥瘕，僻處脅下，將成負固不服之勢，故宜急治。（四）鱉甲煎丸行氣逐血之藥頗多，而不嫌其峻；一日三

33. I.e., from the new moon to the full moon.

34. The identity of "Master Lú" is questionable. It could possibly refer to Lú Wénhuī 盧文輝 (1563-1617), a famous philosopher and adherent of the school of *sān yī jiào* 三一教 , uniting Confucianism, Buddhism, and Daoism. Alternately, it could refer to Lú Rénzōng 仁宗, recorded in the official catalogue of the Táng dynasty as the author of a three-volume text called *Shí Jīng* 食經 (*Classic of Food*).

服，不嫌其急，所謂乘其未集而擊之也。

(1) The qì of heaven completes one cycle of change in fifteen days, and the qì of humans also completes one cycle of change in fifteen days. When the qì changes, the evil should resolve.
(2) If it doesn't, then after thirty days the qì of heaven and of humans completes yet another cycle of change and the evil is naturally unable to lodge.
(3) But if the patient still does not recover in spite of this change, the evil must avail itself of the blood and lean on phlegm, binding to form concretions and conglomerations that hide below the rib-sides. Because this is forming a strategic position with the power to disobey, you should treat immediately.
(4) *Biē Jiǎ Jiān Wán* contains a large number of medicinals that move qì and expel [static] blood, and yet we cannot blame it for [excessive] fierceness. It is to be taken three doses in one day, and yet we cannot blame it for its rashness. This is what is called overwhelming that which has not yet gathered and attacking it.

Quotation by Wáng Jìnsān 王晉三云:

（一）鱉甲煎丸，都用異類靈動之物，若水陸，若飛潛，升者降者，走者伏者，咸備焉。（二）但恐諸虫扰亂神明，取鱉甲為君守之。（三）其泄厥陰破癥瘕之功，有非草木所能比者。（四）阿膠達表熄風，鱉甲入里守神，蜣螂動而性升，蜂房毒可引下，䗪蟲破血，鼠婦走氣，葶藶泄氣閉，大黄泄血閉，赤硝軟堅，桃仁破結，烏扇降厥陰相火，紫葳破厥陰血結，乾薑和陽退寒，黄芩和陰退熱。（五）和表里則有柴胡、桂枝，調營衛則有人參、白芍；厚朴達原，劫去其邪，丹皮入陰，提出其熱，石韋開上焦之水，瞿麦滌下焦之水，半夏和胃而通陰陽，灶灰性溫走氣，清酒性暖走血。（六）統而言之，不越厥陰、陽明二經之藥，故久瘧邪去營衛而着臟腑者，即非瘧母，亦可借以截之。（七）按金匱惟此丸及薯蕷丸藥品最多，皆治正虛邪着久而不去之病，非集血氣之藥，攻補兼施，未易奏功。

(1) *Biē Jiǎ Jiān Wán* uses all ingredients of strange sorts, spirited and moving, whether in the water or on dry land, whether flying or submerged under water, upbearing ones and downbearing ones, running ones and those acting latently, all of them are included in it.
(2) Nevertheless, based on the fear that the various insects might harass and derange the spirit light, [the formula] chooses *biē jiǎ* as the sovereign to guard it.
(3) Its effect of discharging juéyīn and breaking up concretions and conglomerations

cannot be matched by any herbal ingredients.

(4) *Ē jiāo* outthrusts the exterior and extinguishes wind; *biē jiǎ* enters the interior and guards the spirit; *qiāng láng* stirs and is by nature upbearing; *fēng fáng* is able to draw toxins out through precipitation; *zhè chóng* breaks blood; *shǔ fù* penetrates the qì; *tíng lì* discharges blocked qì; *dà huáng* discharges blocked blood; *chì xiāo* softens hardness; *táo rén* breaks up bindings; *wū shàn* downbears ministerial fire in juéyīn; *zǐ wēi* breaks up bound blood in juéyīn; *gān jiāng* harmonizes yáng and abates cold; and *huáng qín* harmonizes yīn and abates heat.

(5) For harmonizing the interior and exterior, we have *chái hú* and *guì zhī*; for balancing construction and defense, we have *rén shēn* and *bái sháo*. *Hòu pò* opens the source and forces the evil out; *mǔ dān pí* enters yīn and lifts out the heat therein; *shí wéi* opens the water in the upper burner; *qū mài* flushes away the water in the lower burner; *bàn xià* harmonizes the stomach and frees the flow of yīn and yáng; stove ashes are warming by nature and penetrate qì; and clear liquor is by nature warm and penetrates the blood.

(6) In conclusion, we can say: Do not skip medicinal substances that treat the two channels of juéyīn and yángmíng. Therefore conditions where prolonged malaria evil has gone into construction and defense and attached itself to the viscera and bowels are in fact not a case of mother of malaria and can be cut short by means of this method.

(7) In the *Jīn Guì Yào Lüè*, only these pills and *Shǔ Yù Wán* have the greatest number of medicinal ingredients and both of them treat conditions of right vacuity and evil chronically adhering and not leaving. These are not medicinals that gather blood and qì, but they have the double action of attack and supplementation. It is not easy to achieve success in this.

白虎加桂枝湯

Bái Hǔ Jiā Guì Zhī Tāng

White Tiger Decoction with Cinnamon Twig Added

治溫瘧者，其脈如平，身無寒但熱，骨節煩疼，時嘔，此湯主之。

A treatment for warm malaria characterized by a pulse that is like normal, a body with no [signs of] cold but only heat, vexing pain in the bones and joints, and occasional retching. This decoction rules.

知母（六兩）石膏（一斤）甘草（二兩，炙）粳米（六合）桂枝（三兩）

zhī mǔ	知母		18g
shí gāo	石膏		48g
gān cǎo	甘草	honey-fried	6g
jīng mǐ	粳米		120ml
guì zhī	桂枝		9g

上五味，以水一斗，煮米熟，湯成去滓，溫服一升，日三服。

Cook the five ingredients above in 2,000ml of water until the rice [*jīng mǐ*] is done. When the decoction is finished, remove the dregs. Take 200ml heated, three doses a day.

Song 歌曰：

白虎原湯論已詳，
桂加三兩另名方；
無寒但熱為溫瘧，
骨節煩疼嘔又妨。
白虎湯歌貝傷寒歌括。

The original White Tiger Decoction has already been discussed in detail.
Of *guì zhī* add nine grams to the so-named formula.

Absence of cold but only heat constitutes warm malaria.
Vexing pain in the bones and joints and retching also hinder.
For the song on White Tiger Decoction, see the *Cháng Shā Fāng Gē Kuò*.

Quotation by Wáng Jìnsān 王晉三云：

（一）內經論瘧，以先熱後寒，邪藏於骨髓者，為溫、癉二瘧。（二）仲景以但熱不寒、邪藏於心者，為溫、癉二瘧。（三）內經所言，是邪之深者；仲景所言，是邪之淺者也。其殆補內經之未逮歟？（四）治以白虎加桂枝湯，方義原在心營肺衛，白虎湯清營分熱邪，加桂枝引領石膏、知母上行至肺，從衛分泄熱，使邪之鬱於表者，頃刻致和而瘧已。（五）至於內經溫、癉瘧，雖未有方，然同是少陰之伏邪。（六）在手經者為實邪，在足經者為虛邪。（七）頭邪尚不發表而用清降，何況虛邪有不顧慮其亡陰者耶？臨證之生心化裁，是所望於用之者矣。

(1) The *Huáng Dì Nèi Jīng* discusses malaria as being characterized by first heat and then cold and by evil hiding in the bones and marrow and refers to two types of malaria, namely warm malaria and *dàn* malaria.[35]
(2) Zhāng Zhòngjǐng describes the two types of warm and pure-heat malaria as being characterized by only heat without any cold and by evil hiding in the heart.
(3) What the *Huáng Dì Nèi Jīng* is talking about is the depth of the evil. What Zhāng Zhòngjǐng is talking about is the shallowness of evil. Is it that he is almost supplementing what the *Huáng Dì Nèi Jīng* has not captured yet?
(4) In the treatment with ***Bái Hǔ Jiā Guì Zhī Tāng***, the meaning of the formula lies originally in heart construction and lung defense. ***Bái Hǔ Tāng*** clears the heat evil in the construction layer and the added ***guì zhī*** leads ***shí gāo*** and ***zhī mǔ*** upward to run into the lung, thereby discharging heat from the defense layer. This causes the condition of evil lying depressed in the exterior to instantly return to harmony and the malaria to subsist.
(5) Now arriving at the question of warm malaria and pure-heat malaria in the *Huáng Dì Nèi Jīng*, although there is not yet a formula attached, it is nevertheless identical to evil lying latent in shàoyīn.
(6) If it is in the hand channel, it is a repletion evil; if it is in the foot channel, it is a vacuity evil.
(7) If evil in the head has not yet effused through the exterior and yet we use clearing and downbearing [treatments], how could we not worry that vacuity evil would lead to yīn collapse? Paying attention and making changes [to the formula] in accordance with the signs means that we look at the application.

35. According to Wiseman terminology, this is translated as pure-heat malaria.

蜀漆散

Shǔ Qī Sǎn

Dichroa Leaf Powder

治瘧多寒者，名曰牝瘧，此散主之。

A treatment for malaria with more [signs of] cold [than of heat], which is called "female malaria". This powder rules it.

蜀漆（燒去腥）雲母（燒二日夜）龍骨（等分）

shǔ qī	蜀漆	roasted until the fishy smell has disappeared
yún mǔ	雲母	roasted for two days and nights
lóng gǔ	龍骨	

上三味杵為散，未發前，以漿水服半錢匕。

Pestle equal parts of the three ingredients above to make a powder. Before the malaria erupts, take half a *qián*-spoon in fermented grain-water.

Song 歌曰：

陽為痰阻伏心間，
牝瘧陰邪自往還；
蜀漆云龍平等杵，
先時漿服不逾閑。

When yáng is affected by phlegm obstruction lying latent in the heart,
In female malaria yīn evil comes and goes all on its own.
Shǔ qī, yún mǔ, and *lóng gǔ* all in equal amounts and pestled,
Take before [an attack] in fermented rice water and [the malaria] will not be more than a trifle.

Quotation by Wáng Jìnsān 王晉三云:

（一）邪氣結伏於心下，心陽鬱遏不舒，瘧發寒多熱少，不可謂其陰寒也。（二）主之以蜀漆散，通心經之陽，開發伏氣而使營衛調和。（三）蜀漆，常山苗也，苗性輕揚，生用能吐；云母在土中，蒸地氣上升而為云，故能入陰分，逐邪外出於表。（四）然邪氣久留心，主之宮城，恐逐邪涌吐，內亂神明，故佐以龍骨鎮心宁神，則吐法轉為和法矣。

(1) When evil qì binds and lies latent below the heart, heart yáng is depressed, obstructed, and constrained, and the malaria erupts with more cold and less heat [signs]. We cannot refer to this as yīn cold.
(2) Ruling it by means of *Shǔ Qī Sǎn* has the effect of freeing the flow of yáng in the heart channel, opening up latent qì and harmonizing construction and defense.
(3) *Shǔ qī* is the sprouts of *cháng shān* and the nature of sprouts is to be light and uplifting. When used raw, it can cause vomiting. *Yún mǔ* is found in the earth. It steams the qì of earth to rise up and form clouds. Therefore it is able to enter the yīn aspect and expel evil by making it exit through the exterior.
(4) Nevertheless, if evil qì has lodged in the heart, the palace of the ruler, for a long time, I fear that expelling evil by inducing gushing vomiting can internally derange the spirit light. Therefore [the other ingredients in the formula] are assisted by *lóng gǔ*, which settles the heart and calms the spirit. As a result, the method of vomiting is turned around into a method of harmonization.

附外台秘要三方

Attached: Three Formulas from the *Wài Tái Mì Yào*[36]

牡蠣湯

Mǔ Lì Tāng

Oyster Shell Decoction

治牡瘧 。

A treatment for male malaria.

牡蠣麻黃（ 各四兩 ）甘草（ 二兩 ）蜀漆（ 三兩 ）

mǔ lì	牡蠣	12g
má huáng	麻黃	12g
gān cǎo	甘草	6g
shǔ qī	蜀漆	9g

（ 一 ）上四味，以水八升，先煮蜀漆 、麻黃，去上沫，得六升 。（ 二 ）內諸藥，煮取二升，溫服一升 。（ 三 ）若吐，則勿更服 。

(1) Of the four ingredients above, first simmer the *shǔ qī* and *má huáng* in 1,600ml of water, removing the foam above, until reduced to 1,200ml.
(2) Add all the other ingredients and simmer until reduced to a 400ml. Take 200ml per dose heated.
(3) If there is vomiting, do not take any more doses.

36. *Essential Secrets from a Border Official/ the Palace Library*, written in 752 CE by Wáng Táo 王燾.

Song 歌曰:

先煎三兩蜀漆四兩麻黃，
四兩牡蠣二甘後煮良；
邪鬱胸中須吐越，
驅寒散結並通陽。

First simmer **nine grams** *shǔ qī* and **twelve grams** *má huáng*,
Then simmer with twelve of *mǔ lì* and six of *gān cǎo*, excellent!
Evil that is depressed in the chest must be surpassed by vomiting,
Expel cold, dissipate bindings, and free the flow of yáng.

Commentary by [Chén] Yuánxī 犀按:

（一）瘧多寒者名牡瘧。（二）是痰飲填塞胸中，阻心陽之氣不得外通故也。

(1) Malaria that is characterized by more cold [than heat] is called male malaria.
(2) It is a condition that is caused by phlegm-rheum stuffing up the chest and obstructing the qì of heart yáng so that it is unable to freely flow to the outside.

Quotation by Master Zhào[37] 趙氏云:

（一）牡蠣軟堅消結；麻黃非獨散寒，且能發越陽氣，使通於外。
（二）結散陽通，其病自愈。

(1) *Mǔ lì* softens hardness and disperses bindings. *Má huáng* not only dissipates cold but is also able to bring yáng qì up and out, causing it to flow freely to the outside.
(2) When bindings are dissipated and yáng is flowing freely, the disease is cured on its own.

37. "Master Zhào" is most likely a reference to Zhào Xiànkě 趙獻可, the author of the *Yī Guàn* 醫貫 (*Thorough Knowledge of Medicine*) published in 1687. He is most famous for his elucidation of the *mìng mén* 命門 (Gate of Life).

柴胡去半夏加栝蔞根湯

Chái Hú Qù Bàn Xià Jiā Guā Lóu Gēn Tāng

Bupleurum Decoction with Pinellia Removed and with Trichosanthes Root Added

治瘧病發渴者，亦治勞瘧 。

A treatment for malaria disease that manifests with thirst when erupting. It also treats taxation malaria.

柴胡（ 八兩 ）人參黃芩甘草（ 各三兩 ）栝蔞根（ 四兩 ）生薑（ 三兩 ）大棗（ 十二枚 ）

chái hú	柴胡	24g
rén shēn	人參	9g
huáng qín	黃芩	9g
gān cǎo	甘草	9g
guā lóu gēn	栝蔞根	12g
shēng jiāng	生薑	9g
dà zǎo	大棗	12 pcs

上七味，以水一斗二升，煮取六升，去滓，再煎，取三升，溫服一升，日三服 。

Simmer the seven ingredients above in 2,400ml of water until reduced to 1,200ml. Remove the dregs and simmer again until reduced to 600ml. Take 200ml per dose heated, three doses a day.

Song 歌曰:

柴胡去夏為傷陰，
加入蔞根四兩珍，
瘧病渴因邪灼液，
蔞根潤燥可生津 。

Use *chái hú* with *bàn xià* removed because it damages yīn,
The addition of twelve grams of *guā lóu gēn* is of great value.
In malaria disease, thirst is caused by evil burning the fluids,
And *guā lóu gēn* moistens dryness and is able to engender liquid.

Quotation by Wáng Jìnsān 王晉三云:

（一）正瘧，寒熱相間，邪發於少陽。與傷寒邪發於少陽者稍異。（二）內經言：夏傷於大暑，秋傷於風，病以時作，名曰寒瘧。（三）金匱云:瘧脈多弦，弦數者風發，正於淒愴之水寒，久伏於湊理皮膚之間，營氣先傷，而後風傷衛。（四）故仲景用柴胡去半夏，而加栝蔞根，其義深且切矣。（五）蓋少陽瘧病發渴者，由風火內淫，劫奪津液而然，奚堪半夏性滑利竅，重傷陰液，故去之。（六）而加天花粉生津潤燥，豈非與正傷寒半表半裡之邪，當用半夏和胃而通陰陽者有別乎?

(1) In regular malaria, cold and heat alternate with each other and the evil erupts in shàoyáng. It is slightly different from the way that evil erupts in shàoyáng in cold damage conditions.
(2) The *Huáng Dì Nèi Jīng* said: "If a person has suffered damage during summer from great summerheat or during fall from wind, and the disease erupts seasonally, this is called 'cold malaria'.
(3) The *Jīn Guì Yào Lüè* said: "The pulse of malaria is predominantly stringlike. If it is stringlike and rapid, it means wind is erupting. In regular malaria, it is the distressingly frigid water cold that is lying latent in the space of the interstices in the skin, as a result of which construction qì is damaged first, and wind subsequently damages the defense.
(4) Therefore Zhāng Zhòngjǐng uses *Chái Hú* [*Tāng*] but without *bàn xià* and with the addition of *guā lóu gēn*. Its meaning is deep as well as penetrating.
(5) Now, when shàoyáng malaria eruptions are accompanied by thirst, it is caused by wind and fire spreading internally and seizing the fluids. How can [such a patient] endure the nature of *bàn xià*, which is slippery and disinhibs the orifices, thereby further damaging the yīn fluids? For this reason, it is removed [from the formula].
(6) How could the addition of *tiān huā fěn*,[38] which engenders fluids and moistens dryness, not be different from straight cold damage conditions where the evil is located half in the exterior and half in the interior, for which you use *bàn xià* to harmonize the stomach and free the flow of yīn and yáng?

38. *Tiān huā fěn* 天花粉 is merely an alternate name for *guā lóu gēn* 栝蔞根 (Root of Trichosanthis kirilowii).

柴胡桂薑湯

Chái Hú Guì Jiāng Tāng

Bupleurum, Cinnamon Twig, and Dried Ginger Decoction

歌見長沙方歌括。

For the song, see the *Cháng Shā Fāng Gē Kuò*.

治瘧寒多微有熱，或但寒不熱，服一劑如神。

A treatment for malaria that manifests with increased cold and slight presence of heat or with only cold and no heat. Taking one preparation will work like magic.

柴胡（半斤）桂枝（三兩）乾薑（二兩）栝蔞根（四兩）黃芩（三兩）甘草（二兩）牡蠣（二兩）

chái hú	柴胡	24g
guì zhī	桂枝	9g
gān jiāng	乾薑	6g
guā lóu gēn	栝蔞根	12g
huáng qín	黃芩	9g
gān cǎo	甘草	6g
mǔ lì	牡蠣	6g

（一）上七味，以水一斗，煮取六升。（二）去滓，再煎，取三升，溫服一升，日三。（三）初服微煩，復服汗出便愈。

(1) Simmer the seven ingredients above in 2,000ml of water until reduced to 1,000ml.
(2) Remove the dregs and simmer again until reduced to 500ml. Take 200ml per dose heated, three doses a day.
(3) If there is mild vexation after the first dose and sweating after the second dose, it means recovery.

Quotation by Wáng Jìnsān 王晉三云:

（一）夏月暑邪，先傷在內之伏陰，至秋復感涼風，更傷衛陽。（二）其瘧寒多微有熱，顯然陰陽無爭，故瘧邪從衛氣行陰二十五度；內無捍格之狀，是營衛俱病矣，故和其陽即當和其陰。（三）用柴胡和少陽之陽，即用黃芩和里；用桂枝和太陽之陽，即用牡蠣和里；用乾薑和陽明之陽，即用天花粉和里；使以甘草調和陰陽。（四）其分兩陽分獨重柴胡者，以正瘧不离乎少陽也；陰藥獨重於花粉者，陰虧之瘧以救液為急務也。（五）和之得其當，故一劑如神。

(1) Summerheat evil in the summer months first damages latent yīn on the inside. Arriving at fall, if [the patient] further contracts cool wind, this additionally damages defensive yáng.
(2) In this kind of malaria, you see increased cold and slight presence of heat, and it is obvious that yīn and yáng are not struggling with each other. Therefore the malaria evil follows the defensive qì and moves in yīn by twenty-five measures. The appearance that there is no resistance on the inside means that construction and defense are both affected by the disease. Therefore harmonizing the patient's yáng must also include harmonizing the patient's yīn.
(3) When you use *chái hú* to harmonize the yáng in shàoyáng, also use *huáng qín* to harmonize the interior. When you use *guì zhī* to harmonize the yáng in tàiyáng, also use *mǔ lì* to harmonize the interior. When you use *gān jiāng* to harmonize the yáng in yángmíng, also use *tiān huā fěn*[39] to harmonize the interior. Allow *gān cǎo* to balance and harmonize yīn and yáng.
(4) The formula singularly emphasizes *chái hú* in its division into the two yáng aspects because regular malaria never leaves shàoyáng. The formula focuses on *tiān huā fěn* alone among the yīn medicinals, because in malaria when yīn is depleted, rescuing the fluids is the most urgent task.
(5) This formula harmonizes these [strategies] in such a way that each is treated appropriately. Therefore even a single preparation works like magic.

Quotation by a sage from the past 先賢云:

（一）瘧病不離少陽，少陽居半表半裡之間，邪入與陰爭則寒，出與陽爭則熱。（二）爭則病作，息則病止。（三）止後其邪仍居於少陽之經。（四）愚意外為陽，內為陰。（五）先寒者，邪欲出，其氣干於太陽，衝動寒水之氣而作也。後熱者，以胃為燥土，脾為濕土，濕

39. See note 38 above.

從燥化，則木亦從其化，故為熱為汗也。（六）汗後木邪仍伏於陽明之中，應期而發者，土主信也，蓋久瘧胃虛，得補可愈，故先君用白朮生薑湯多效。

(1) Malaria does not leave shàoyáng, and shàoyáng resides in the space of half exterior and half interior. When the evil enters and struggles with yīn, there is cold. When it exits and struggles with yáng, there is heat.
(2) When there is struggle, the disease erupts. When there is rest, the disease stops.
(3) After stopping, the evil lodges in the shàoyáng channel.
(4) In my humble opinion, outside means yáng and inside means yīn.
(5) The reason that cold comes first is that the evil wants to exit and its qì is interfering with tàiyáng. Surging at and stirring the qì of cold and water, [the malaria] erupts. The reason that heat comes afterwards is that the stomach is dry earth while the spleen is damp earth. Dampness follows dryness and transforms, and hence wood also follows its transformation. Therefore we see heat and we see sweating.
(6) After sweating, the wood evil lies latent in yángmíng. The reason it erupts according to certain times is that earth rules trust. Now in prolonged malaria the stomach becomes vacuous. When it receives supplementation, [the malaria] can be cured. For this reason, the gentleman from the past used *Bái Zhú Shēng Jiāng Tāng* with great results.

中風歷節方
Zhòng Fēng Lì Jié Fāng

Formulas for Wind Strike and Joint-Running

侯氏黑散
Hóu Shì Hēi Sǎn
Master Hóu's Black Powder

治大風四肢煩重，心中惡寒不足者 。

A treatment for great wind with vexation and heaviness in the four limbs, and in the heart aversion to cold and insufficiency.

菊花（ 四十分 ）白朮 防風（ 各十分 ）桔梗（ 八分 ）黄芩（ 五分 ）細辛 乾薑 人參 茯苓 當歸 川芎 牡蠣 礬石 桂枝（ 各三分 ）

jú huā	菊花	30g
bái zhú	白朮	7.5g
fáng fēng	防風	7.5g
jié gěng	桔梗	6g
huáng qín	黄芩	3.75g
xì xīn	細辛	2.25g
gān jiāng	乾薑	2.25g
rén shēn	人參	2.25g
fú líng	茯苓	2.25g
dāng guī	當歸	2.25g
chuān xiōng	川芎	2.25g
mǔ lì	牡蠣	2.25g
fán shí	礬石	2.25g
guì zhī	桂枝	2.25g

（ 一 ）上十四味，杵為散，酒服方寸匕，日一服 。（ 二 ）初服二十日，溫酒調服 。（ 三 ）禁一切魚肉大蒜等，常宜冷食，六十日止，即藥積在腹中不下也 。（ 四 ）熱食即下矣，冷食自能助藥力 。

(1) Pestle the fourteen ingredients above to process them into a powder and take one gram with liquor, one dose per day.
(2) Initially take [the formula] for twenty days mixed into heated liquor.
(3) All fish, meat, garlic and the like are contraindicated. It is suitable to regularly eat cooling foods. After sixty days, stop. At this time, the medicine has accumulated in the abdomen without being precipitated.
(4) Hot foods will precipitate the medicine! Cool foods are naturally able to assist the strength of the medicine.

Song 歌曰：

黑散辛苓歸桂芎，
參薑礬蠣各三同，
菊宜四十朮防十，
桔八芩須五分通 。

Black powder, with *xì xīn, fú líng, dāng guī, guì zhī, chuān xiōng,*
Rén shēn, gān jiāng, fán shí, mǔ lì, each of them in the amount of two-and-a-quarter grams;
Of *jú huā* thirty grams, of *bái zhú* and *fáng fēng* seven-and-a-half grams;
Of *jié gěng* six and of *huáng qín* three-and-three-quarters grams are required to free the flow.

Quotation by Wáng Jìnsān 王晉三云：

（一）程雲來謂金匱侯氏黑散，系宋人校正附入唐人之方，因逸之，其辨論頗詳。（二）而喻嘉言獨贊其立方之妙，驅風補虛，行堵截之法，良非思議可到。（三）方中取用礬石以固澀諸藥，冷服四十日，使之留積不散，以漸填其空竅，則風自熄而不生矣。（四）此段議論，獨開千古之秘，誠為治中風之要旨。（五）讀方下云，初服二十日，用溫酒調，是不欲其遽填也；後服六十日，並禁熱食，則一任填空竅矣。（六）夫填竅本之內經久塞其空，是謂良工之語，煞有來歷。

(1) According to Chéng Yúnlái,[40] ***Hóu Shì Hēi Sǎn*** from the *Jīn Guì Yào Lüè* is actually a *Táng* period formula that was added by the *Sòng* editors during correction. Because he regarded it as extraneous, his debate on this issue is very detailed.
(2) And yet Yù Jiāyán[41] is the only one to praise the subtlety with which this formula has been created, driving out wind and supplementing vacuity to carry out the method of blocking and interrupting [the invasion of wind]. It is so skillfull that no rational thought can reach it.
(3) In the formula, we use ***fán shí*** to secure and astringe all the other medicinals, and [after the first twenty days] take it with cool [food and drink] for forty days to cause it to collect without dispersing. Thereby it slowly fills in the orifices so that wind is extinguished on its own and will not be generated further!
(4) Discussing this section alone opens up a secret from a thousand antiquities and truly is the key to treating wind strike.
(5) When reading the formula, further below it includes the instruction for the first twenty days to take it mixed into heated liquor. The reason for this is that you do not want to fill in [the orifices] too rapidly. The prohibition against hot foods during the subsequent sixty days of taking it allows [the medicine] to fill in the empty orifices!
(6) Now the root of filling in the orifices, namely the phrase "stopping up their emptiness for a long time" from the *Huáng Dì Nèi Jīng*, is the language of a skilled craftsperson and has great historical precedence.

---

40. A famous physician from the eighteenth century who specialized in Cold Damage treatments.

41. A colleague and contemporary of Chéng Yúnlái's who answered his questions on Cold Damage.
Yù Jiāyán (1585-1664) was a failed government official who became a monk at the age of 50 and devoted himself to the study of Buddhism and medicine. Several years later, after realizing his skills as a physician, he left the monastic life and became a professional physician. Late in life, he became so famous for his skills as a physician that he is known as one of the three great masters of the early *Qīng* dynasty.

風引湯

Fēng Yǐn Tāng

Wind-Pulling Decoction

除熱癱癎，主大人風引，少小驚癎瘈瘲，日數發，醫所不療，除熱方 。巢氏云:腳氣宜此湯 。

[A treatment] to eliminate heat paralysis and epilepsy. Ruling wind-pulling in adults as well as pediatric fright epilepsy with tugging and slackening, with several attacks a day, which the doctors are unable to cure, this is a formula for eliminating heat. As Master Cháo[42] said, this formula is also suitable [as a treatment] for leg qì.[43]

大黃 乾薑 龍骨（ 各四兩 ）桂枝（ 三兩 ）甘草 牡蠣（ 各二兩 ）寒水石 滑石 赤石脂 白石脂 紫石英 石膏（ 各六兩）

dà huáng	大黃	12g
gān jiāng	乾薑	12g
lóng gǔ	龍骨	12g
guì zhī	桂枝	9g
gān cǎo	甘草	6g
mǔ lì	牡蠣	6g
hán shuǐ shí	寒水石	18g
huá shí	滑石	18g
chì shí zhī	赤石脂	18g
bái shí zhī	白石脂	18g

42. This is most likely a reference to Cháo Yuánfāng 巢元方, the famous author of the *Zhū Bìng Yuán Hòu Lùn* who lived in the seventh century.

43. Leg qì is a disease name that is explained in the *Zhǒu Hòu Bèi Jí Fāng* 肘後備急方 *Prescriptions [to Carry] Behind the Elbow* by Gě Hóng 葛洪. It is caused by external contraction of dampness evil or wind toxin or by rich-flavored food and drink. Accumulating dampness engenders heat, which pours into the legs and causes disease. In terms of symptoms, you first see numbness, soreness, weakness and lack of strength in the legs, possibly cramps, swelling, withering, and heat effusion. When it enters the abdomen and attacks the heart, you see discomfort in the lower abdomen, vomiting and lack of appetite, heart palpitations, oppression in the chest, panting, a muddled spirit, and confused speech.

zǐ shí yīng	紫石英	18g
shí gāo	石膏	18g

上十二味，杵，粗篩，以葦囊盛之，取三指撮，井花水三升，煮三沸，溫服一升。

Pestle the twelve ingredients above and strain through a coarse sieve. Put it in a purse made out of reeds [for storage]. Take a three-finger pinch and simmer it in 600ml of water drawn from a well first thing in the morning, bringing it to a boil three times. Take 200ml per dose heated.[44]

Song 歌曰:

四兩大黃二牡甘，
龍薑四兩桂枝三，
滑寒赤白紫膏六，
癱癇諸風個里探。

Twelve grams of *dà huáng*, six grams of *mǔ lì* and *gān cǎo*;
Of *lóng gǔ* and *gān jiāng* twelve grams each, of *guì zhī* nine grams;
Of *huá shí, hán shuǐ shí, chì shí zhī, bái shí zhī, zǐ shí yīng* and *shí gāo* eighteen grams each;
Paralysis and epilepsy and the various [forms of] wind, each are detected in the interior.

Commentary by [Chén] Yuánxī 元犀按:

（一）大人中風牽引，小兒驚癇瘈瘲，正火熱生風，五臟亢盛，及其歸逆入心，其治同也。（二）此方用大黃為君，以蕩滌風火熱濕之邪；隨用乾薑之止而不行者以補之；用佳枝、甘草以緩其勢；又用石藥之澀以堵其路；而石藥之中又取滑石、石膏清金以平其木；赤白石脂厚土以除其濕；龍骨、牡蠣以斂其精神魂魄之紛馳；用寒水石以助腎之真陰，不為陽光所劫；更用紫石英以補心神之虛，恐心不明而十二經危也。（三）明此以治入臟之風，游刃有余矣。（四）後人以石藥過多而棄之，昧孰甚焉！

(1) The treatment of wind strike with stretching and pulling, of pediatric fright epilepsy with tugging and slackening, and of ordinary fire-heat engendering wind that exuberates

44. A note by historical editors of this text states: It is good to reduce the *gān jiāng* and *guì zhī* in this formula by half.

in the viscera and then turns around to enter the heart, is identical.
(2) This formula uses *dà huáng* as the sovereign, to flush out the evil of wind, fire, heat, and dampness. Next, it uses *gān jiāng* for its effect of stopping movement rather then inducing it, in order to supplement. It uses *guì zhī* and *gān cǎo* to moderate the force [of the disease]. And moreover uses the astringency of the stone medicinals to fill up its path. Among the medicinal stones, it uses *huá shí* and *shí gāo* to clear metal and thereby calm wood; it uses *chì shí zhī* and *bái shí zhī* to thicken earth and thereby eliminate dampness; it uses *lóng gǔ* and *mǔ lì* to restrain the spirit and the *hún* and *pò* souls from all galloping after each other; it uses *hán shuǐ shí* to assist the true yīn in the kidney so that it is not plundered by the light of yáng; and it uses *zǐ shí yīng* to supplement the vacuity of the heart spirit, because we fear that if the heart is not clear the twelve channels are at risk.
(3) When you understand these [actions] and thereby treat wind that has entered the viscera, you can wield the butcher's knife with more than adequate skill.[45]
(4) In later times, people have abandoned this formula because of the excessive use of stone medicinals [in this formula], but what blindness could be greater than that!

45. An expression meaning that you are more than adequately equipped for the task at hand.

防己地黄湯
Fáng Jǐ Dì Huáng Tāng
Fángjǐ and Rehmannia Decoction

治中風，病如狂狀，妄行，獨語不休，無熱，其脈浮者。

A treatment for wind strike, when the disease looks like mania, with senseless actions and talking to oneself without stopping, absence of heat, and a floating pulse.

防己甘草（各一分）桂枝防風（各三分）

fáng jǐ	防己	0.75g
gān cǎo	甘草	0.75g
guì zhī	桂枝	2.25g
fáng fēng	防風	2.25g

（一）上四味，以酒一杯漬之，絞取汁。（二）生地黄二斤，㕮咀，蒸之如斗米飯久。（三）以銅器盛藥汁，更絞地黄汁，和，分再服。

(1) Soak the four ingredients above in one cup of liquor and squeeze out to get the juice.
(2) Pound ninety-six grams of *shēng dì huáng* and steam it for the length of time it takes to cook a dipper-full of rice.
(3) Fill a copper vessel with the juice from the medicinals. Also squeeze out the juice from the *dì huáng* and combine with that. Divide and take in two doses.

Song 歌曰:

妄行獨語病如狂，
一分己甘三桂防，
杯酒淋來取清汁，
二斤蒸地絞和嘗。

Senseless actions and talking to oneself, a condition like mania:
Three-quarters-of-a gram of *fáng jǐ* and *gān cǎo* and two-and-a-quarter grams of *guì zhī* and *fáng fēng*.
Soak them in a cup of liquor and remove the clear juice.
Squeeze out ninety-six grams of steamed *dì huáng* and taste them together.

Quotation by Xú Língtāi[46] 徐靈胎云:

（一）生漬取清汁歸之於陽，以散邪熱；蒸取濃汁歸之於陰，以養血。（二）此皆治風邪歸并於心，而為癲癇惊狂之病。與中風，風痹自當另看。

(1) [Preparing medicinals by] using them fresh, soaking them, and taking the clear juice makes them return to yáng, thereby dispersing evil heat; using then steamed and taking the concentrated juice makes them return to yīn, thereby nourishing blood.
(2) All of these treat wind evil that has returned to merge with the heart and is causing conditions of epilepsy, fright, and mania. For wind strike and wind impediment, you should naturally look elsewhere.

46. Xú Língtāi (1693-1771), also known as Xú Dàchūn 徐大椿, was a famous polymath and scholar-physician from the *Qīng* dynasty who published a profusion of books on medicine, including a collection of case histories.

頭風摩散
Tóu Fēng Mó Sǎn
Head Wind Rubbing Powder

治頭風 。

A treatment for head wind.

大附子（ 一枚 ）鹽（ 等分 ）

dà fù zǐ	大附子	1 pc
salt	鹽	equal amounts

上二味為散 。沐了，以方寸匕摩頭上，令藥力行 。

Process the two ingredients above into a powder. After washing the patient's hair, rub a gram [of the powder] into the top of the patient's head so that the power of the medicine is activated.

Song 歌曰：

頭風偏痛治如何？
附子和鹽等分摩；
軀殼病生須外治，
馬膏桑引亦同科 。

How do you treat head wind with unilateral pain?
By rubbing on *fù zǐ* and salt in equal amounts.
When disease arises in the shell of the body, you must treat it externally.
Horse fat and mulberry [hook] pulling are also in the same category [of treatments].

（一）靈樞：馬膏，白酒和桂，桑鉤鉤之。（二）醇酒入椒、薑，綿絮熨之，三十遍而止。（三）皆外法也。特於此推論之。

(1) The *Líng Shū* mentions horse fat, white liquor mixed with *guì zhī* [powder], and using a hook made of mulberry [wood] to "hook" [the wind].[47]
(2) Make a hot compress of silk padding with fine wine prepared with *shǔ jiāo* and *gān jiāng*. Press it on thirty times and then stop.
(3) All of these are external treatments. They are discussed by inference here specifically for this [condition].

47. This passage is found in *Líng Shū* chapter 13.

桂枝芍藥知母湯

Guì Zhī Sháo Yào Zhī Mǔ Tāng

Cinnamon Twig, Peony, and Anemarrhena Decoction

治諸肢節疼痛，身體尪羸，腳腫如脫，頭眩短氣，溫溫欲吐者 。

A treatment for all pain in the joints of the extremities, with lameness and emaciation of the body, swelling in the feet as in desertion, dizziness in the head and shortness of breath, a feeling of uncomfortable warmth and being on the verge of vomiting.

桂枝（ 四兩 ）芍藥（ 三兩 ）甘草 麻黃 附子（ 各二兩 ）白朮 知母 防風（ 各四兩 ）生薑（ 五兩 ）

guì zhī	桂枝	12g
sháo yào	芍藥	9g
gān cǎo	甘草	6g
má huáng	麻黃	6g
fù zǐ	附子	6g
bái zhú	白朮	12g
zhī mǔ	知母	12g
fáng fēng	防風	12g
shēng jiāng	生薑	15g

上九味，以水七升，先煮麻黃減二升，去上沫 。內諸藥同煎取二升，溫服七合，日三服 。

Of the nine ingredients above, first simmer the *má huáng* in 1,400ml of water until reduced by 400ml. Remove the foam from the top. Add all the other medicinals and simmer in the same way until reduced to 400ml. Take 140ml per dose heated, three doses per day.

Song 歌曰：

腳腫身羸欲吐形，
芍三薑五是前型，
知防朮桂均須四，
附子麻甘二兩停 。

For swelling in the feet, an emaciated body, and being on the verge of vomiting,
Nine grams of *sháo yào* and fifteen grams of *shēng jiāng* are for the type above,
Of *zhī mŭ, fáng fēng, bái zhú,* and *guì zhī,* you must use twelve grams each,
But with *fù zǐ* , *má huáng* and *gān cǎo,* stop at six grams.

Commentary by [Chén] Yuánxī 元犀按：

（一）用桂枝湯去棗加麻黃，以助其通陽。（二）加白朮、防風，以伸其脾氣。（三）加附子、知母，以調其陰陽。（四）多用生薑，以平其嘔逆。

(1) In the application of *Guì Zhī Tāng,* remove *dà zǎo* but add *má huáng* to assist in its action of freeing the flow of yáng.
(2) Add *bái zhú* and *fáng fēng* to stretch the patient's spleen qì.
(3) Add *fù zǐ* and *zhī mŭ* to harmonize the patient's yīn and yáng.
(4) And use a larger amount of *shēng jiāng* to calm the retching counterflow.

烏頭湯

Wū Tóu Tāng

Aconite Main Tuber Decoction

治歷節病不可屈伸疼痛者，又主腳疼痛不可屈伸。

A treatment for joint-running disease that manifest with inability to bend or stretch and pain. [This formula] also rules pain in the feet with inability to bend or stretch them.

麻黃芍藥黃芪甘草（各三兩，炙）烏頭（五枚）

má huáng	麻黃		9g
sháo yào	芍藥		9g
huáng qí	黃芪		9g
gān cǎo	甘草	honey-fried	9g
wū tóu	烏頭		5 pcs

（一）上將烏頭㕮咀，以蜜二升，煎取一升，即出烏頭。（二）另四味，以水三升，煮取一升，去滓。（三）內蜜煎中，更煎之，服七合。（四）不知，盡服之。

(1) Of the above ingredients, take the *wū tóu* and pound it. Then stew it in 400ml of honey until reduced to 200ml. Remove the *wū tóu*.
(2) Simmer the other four ingredients in 600ml of water until reduced to 200ml and remove the dregs.
(3) Add the honey brew to this and stew it again. Take 140ml per dose.
(4) If you do not notice a change, take the rest [of the decoction].

Song 歌曰:

歷節疼來不屈伸，
或加腳氣痛維均，
芍芪麻草皆三兩，
五粒烏頭煮蜜勻。

For joint-running with pain that comes with inability bend or stretch,
Possibly with the addition of leg qì pain evenly linked,
Sháo yào, huáng qí, má huáng, and *gān cǎo,* all in the amount of nine grams,
Five small pieces of *wū tóu* simmered in honey and well blended in.

Quotation by Yóu Zàijīng 尤在涇云:

（一）此治寒濕歷節之正法也。（二）寒濕之邪，非麻黃、烏頭不能去；而病在筋節，又非皮毛之邪，可一汗而散者。（三）故以黃芪之補，白芍之平，甘草之緩，牽制二物。（四）俾得深入而去留邪，如衛瓘監鍾、鄧入蜀，使其成功而不及於亂，乃制方之要妙也。

(1) This formula is the correct method for treating cold-damp joint-running.
(2) Without *má huáng* and *wū tóu,* it is impossible to get rid of the evil of cold-damp. And this disease is one that is located in the sinews and joints and not one associated with an evil of the skin and hair, which can simply be removed by sweating alone.
(3) Therefore the formula uses the supplementing action of *huáng qí,* the calming action of *bái sháo,* and the moderating action of *gān cǎo* to lead and control these two substances.
(4) These additions allow the formula to enter deeply and remove the lodged evil, just like Wèi Guàn guarded himself as Zhōng and Dèng entered Shǔ, allowing him to be successful instead of being involved in their upheavals.[48] Now this is the key subtlety of preparing this formula.

48. Wèi Guàn (220-291) was a loyal general for the kingdom of Wèi 魏 during the period of the Three Kingdoms who refused to participate in a failed rebellion led by Zhōng and Dèng.

礬石湯

Fán Shí Tāng

Alum Decoction

治脚氣衝心。

A treatment for leg qì surging up against the heart.

礬石（二兩）

fán shí 礬石 6g

上一味，以漿水一斗五升，煎三五沸，浸脚良。

Simmer the single ingredient above in 3,000ml of fermented grain-water, bringing it to a boil three to five times. Soak the feet [in this decoction] for excellent [results].

Song 歌曰：

脚氣衝心礬石湯，
煮須漿水浸之良；
濕收毒解兼除熱，
補卻靈樞外法彰。

For leg qì surging up against the heart use *Fán Shí Tāng*.
Simmer [*fán shí*] in fermented grain-water and then soak [the feet] in this for excellent [results].
[As a result,] dampness disappears, toxins are resolved, and at the same time heat is eliminated.
This formula supplements indeed the exterior methods displayed in the *Líng Shū*.

Quotation by Yóu Zàijīng 尤在涇云：

（一）脚氣之病，濕傷於下而氣衝於上。（二）礬石味酸澀性燥，能卻水，收濕，解毒，毒解濕收，上衝自止。

(1) In the disease of leg qì, dampness afflicts damage in the lower body and qì surges into the upper body.
(2) The flavor of *fán shí* is sour and astringent, its nature is dry. It is able to eliminate water, make dampness disappear, and resolve toxins. When toxins are resolved and dampness has disappeared, the upsurging stops on its own.

附方

Fù Fāng

Attached Formulas

古今錄驗續命湯

Gŭ Jīn Lù Yàn Xù Mìng Tāng

Continuing-Life Decoction from the *Gŭ Jīn Lù Yàn*[49]

治中風痱，身體不能自收持，口不能言，冒昧不知痛處，或拘急不得轉側 。

A treatment for wind strike with prickly heat, inability to contract and hold together the body, inability to speak, veiling and confusion so that the patient does not know the location of the pain, and possibly hypertonicity and inability to turn to the side.

麻黃 桂枝 人參 甘草 乾薑 石膏 當歸（ 各三兩 ）川芎（ 一兩五錢 ）杏仁（ 四十枚 ）

má huáng	麻黃	9g
guì zhī	桂枝	9g
rén shēn	人參	9g
gān cǎo	甘草	9g
gān jiāng	乾薑	9g
shí gāo	石膏	9g
dāng guī	當歸	9g
chuān xiōng	川芎	4.5g
xìng rén	杏仁	40 pits

49. *Gŭ Jīn Lù Yàn* 古今錄驗 (*Records of Experiences from the Past and Present*) is an early formula collection that is quoted in such medieval formularies as the *Wài Tái Mì Yào*, *Bèi Jí Qiān Jīn Yào Fāng* and *Yī Xīn Fāng* 醫心方 (*Prescriptions from the Heart of Medicine*). It is first mentioned in the official catalogue of the early *Táng* dynasty as a text in 50 scrolls. Author and exact date of publication are unknown and the text as a whole is lost.

（一）上九味，以水一斗，煮取四升，溫服一升。（二）當小汗，薄覆脊，憑几坐。（三）汗出則愈；不汗，更服。（四）無所禁，勿當風。（五）並治但伏不得臥，咳逆上氣，面目浮腫。

(1) Simmer the nine ingredients above in 2,000ml of water until reduced to 800ml. Take 200ml per dose, heated.
(2) The patient should sweat a little. Cover the back with a thin blanket and have them sit up, leaning against a small bench.
(3) If there is sweating, this means recovery. If there is no sweating, take another dose.
(4) [This treatment] has no contraindications, except that you must avoid exposure to wind.
(5) [With this method,] you also treat patients who can only lie face down, but not on their back, cough with counterflow ascent of qì, and puffy swelling in the face and eyes.

Song 歌曰:

薑歸參桂草膏麻，
三兩均勻切莫差，
四十杏仁芎兩半，
古今錄驗主風邪。

With *gān jiāng, dāng guī, rén shēn, guì zhī, gān cǎo, shí gāo,* and *má huáng,*
Nine grams of each of these, blended well with none of them missing,
Forty pits of *xìng rén* and four-and-a-half grams of *chuān xiōng,*
The *Gŭ Jīn Lù Yàn* rules wind evil.

Commentary by [Chén] Yuánxī 元犀按:

（一）風，陽邪也。氣通於肝。痱，閉也。（二）風入閉塞其毛竅，阻滯榮衛不行也。（三）蓋風多挾寒，初中時由皮膚而入，以漸而深入於內，鬱久則化熱，熱則傷陰，陰傷內無以養其臟腑，外不能充於形骸。（四）此即身體不能自收持，口不能言，冒昧不知痛處所由來也。（五）主以古今錄驗續命湯者，取其祛風走表，安內攘外，旋轉上下也。（六）方中麻黃、佳枝、乾薑、杏仁、石膏、甘草，以發其肌表之風邪，兼理其內蘊之熱。（七）又以人參、當歸、川芎補血調氣，領麻黃、石膏等藥穿筋骨，通經絡，調榮衛，出肌表之邪。（八）是則此方從內達外，圜轉周身，驅邪開痱，無有不到。（九）稱曰古今錄驗續命湯，其命名豈淺哉？

(1) Wind is a yáng evil. Its qì flows to the liver. Prickly heat means blockage.
(2) Wind enters and blocks the person's orifices and body hair and obstructs construction and defense without moving.
(3) Now wind oftentimes is complicated by cold. When it first strikes, it enters through the skin, and then gradually enters deeper into the interior. After it lies there depressed for a long time, it transforms into heat, and the heat subsequently damages yīn. When yīn is damaged, there is nothing in the interior to nourish the person's viscera and bowels and the body is unable on the outside to fill the physical form.
(4) If this situation occurs, then we see inability of the body to contract and hold together, inability to speak, and veiling and confusion so that the person does not know where the pain is coming from.
(5) Ruling this condition with *Xù Mìng Tāng* from the *Gǔ Jīn Lù Yàn* means that you take advantage of its effects of driving out wind and penetrating the exterior, pacifying the inside and resisting [invading evils] on the outside, and cycles all throughout in both the upper and lower body.
(6) In the formula, *má huáng, guì zhī, gān jiāng, xìng rén, shí gāo* and *gān cǎo* are used to effuse the wind evil from the fleshy exterior as well as rectifying the heat smoldering on the inside.
(7) Furthermore, [the formula] uses *rén shēn, dāng guī,* and *chuān xiōng* to supplement blood and balance qì, to lead the medicinals *má huáng, shí gāo,* etc. to penetrate to the sinews and bones, to free the flow in the channels and network vessels, to balance construction and defense, and to discharge evil from the fleshy exterior.
(8) As a result, this formula outthrusts from the inside, cycles all throughout in the entire body, expels evil and opens up prickly heat, reaching every nook and cranny of the body.
(9) How could there be anything frivolous about the name "Continuing-Life Decoction" from the *Gǔ Jīn Lù Yàn*?

千金三黃湯

Qiān Jīn Sān Huáng Tāng

Three Yellows Decoction from the *Bèi Jí Qiān Jīn Yào Fāng*

治中風，手足拘急，百節疼痛，煩熱心亂，惡寒，經日不欲飲食。

A treatment for wind strike with hypertonicity in the hands and feet, pain in the hundred joints, vexing heat and derangement in the heart, aversion to cold, and no desire for food or drink for a number of days.

麻黃（五分）獨活（四分）細辛（二分）黃芪（二分）黃芩（三分）

má huáng	麻黃	3.75g
dú huó	獨活	3g
xì xīn	細辛	1.5g
huáng qí	黃芪	1.5g
huáng qín	黃芩	2.25g

（一）上五味，以水六升，煮取二升，分溫三服。（二）一服小汗，二服大汗。（三）心熱加大黃二分，腹滿加枳實一枚，氣逆加人參三分，悸加牡蠣三分，渴加栝蔞根三分，先有寒加附子一枝。

(1) Simmer the five ingredients above in 1,200ml of water until reduced to 400ml. Divide and take heated in three doses.
(2) After one dose, there will be mild sweating, after two doses great sweating.
(3) For heat in the heart, add one-and-a-half grams of *dà huáng*. For abdominal fullness, add one piece of *zhǐ shí*. For qì counterflow, add two-and-a-quarter grams of *rén shēn*. For palpitations, add two-and-a-quarter grams of *mǔ lì*. For thirst, add two-and-a-quarter grams of *guā lóu gēn*. For presence of cold beforehand, add one piece of *fù zǐ*.

Song 歌曰:

風乘火勢亂心中，
節痛肢拘絡不通；
二分芪辛四分獨，
黃芩三分五麻攻 。

For wind overwhelming the force of fire, causing derangement in the heart,
Joint pain, hypertonicity in the limbs, and lack of free flow in the network vessels,
One-and-a-half grams of *huáng qí* and *xì xīn* and three grams of *dú huó*,
Two-and-a-quarter grams of *huáng qín* and three-and-three-quarters of *má huáng* to attack [this condition].

Song for Modifications 加減歌曰:

二分黃加心熱端，
消除腹滿枳枚單，
虛而氣逆宜參補，
牡蠣潛陽悸可安，
增入蔞根能止渴，
各加三分效堪觀，
病前先有寒邪在，
附子一枚仔細看 。

Add one-and-a-half grams of *dà huáng* for extreme heat in the heart;
To disperse abdominal fullness, a single piece of *zhǐ shí*;
For vacuity and counterflow qì, it is appropriate to supplement with *rén shēn*;
Mǔ lì subdues yáng and palpitations can be quieted.
Adding *guā lóu gēn* is able to stop thirst;
Two-and-a-quarter grams of each, and the efficacy is truly spectacular.
If there was cold evil present before the disease,
For one piece of *fù zǐ* look carefully.

Commentary by [Chén] Yuánxī 元犀按:

（一）此附子治風中太少，通護陰陽，驅邪之方也。（二）足太陰屬脾，主四肢，手足拘急，惡寒。（三）經日不欲飲食者，脾不運也。（四）手少陰屬心，主神，心病則神昏，故心亂而發煩熱也。（五）足少陰屬腎，主筋骨，病則百節疼痛也。（六）方用麻黃、黃芪入太陰，宣陽發表，淨脾中之邪。以黃芩清其心熱以止煩，又用細辛、獨活入腎，穿筋骨，以散腎邪，此主治之大意也。（七）方下氣逆加人參等六法，其意未會，不敢強解，留俟後之學者。

(1) This is a formula for conditions where *fù zǐ* as a treatment for wind strike is too little, by freeing the flow of and protecting yīn and yáng, and by driving out evil.
(2) Foot tàiyīn belongs to the spleen and governs the four limbs. [Spleen disease results in] hypertonicity in the hands and feet and aversion to cold.
(3) When you see no desire for food or drink for a number of days, it means that the spleen is not moving [substances throughout the body].
(4) The hand shàoyīn belongs to the heart and governs the spirit. Heart disease results in clouded spirit, therefore we see derangement in the heart and attacks of vexing heat.
(5) The foot shàoyīn belongs to the kidney and governs the sinew and bones. [Kidney] disease results in pain in the hundred joints.
(6) The formula uses *má huáng* and *huáng qí* to enter tàiyīn, perfuse yáng and effuse the exterior, and purge the evil from the spleen. It uses *huáng qín* to clear the heat in the heart and thereby stops the vexation. It furthermore uses *xì xīn* and *dú huó* to enter the kidney and penetrate to the sinews and bones, to dissipate evil from the kidney. This is the general idea behind this treatment.
(7) As for the six methods of adding *rén shēn* for qì counterflow etc. that follow the formula, I do not yet grasp their significance and do not dare to offer forced explanations. Hence I leave them to wait for later scholars.

近效朮附湯

Jìn Xiào Zhú Fù Tāng

White Atractylodes and Aconite Decoction from the *Jìn Xiào Fāng*[50]

治風虛頭重眩，苦極不知食味。暖肌補中，益精氣。

A treatment for wind vacuity with heaviness and dizziness in the head and bitter pain that is so extreme that the patient does not know the flavor of food. It warms the flesh, supplements the center, and boosts essence and qì.

白朮（二兩）附子（一枚半，炮去皮）甘草（一兩，炙）

bái zhú	白朮		6g
fù zǐ	附子	blast-fried, skin removed	1.5 pcs
gān cǎo	甘草	honey-fried	3g

上三味，銼。每五錢匕，生薑五片，大棗一枚，水盞半，煎七分，去滓，溫服。

Grate the three ingredients above. For each [preparation], take five *qián*-spoons full, five slices of *shēng jiāng,* and one piece of *dà zǎo,* and simmer in half a cup of water until reduced to seven tenths. Remove the dregs and take it heated.

50. The *Jìn Xiào Fāng* 近效方 (*Formulas of Intimate Efficacy*) is a now lost formula collection that is frequently quoted in medieval medical texts like the *Wài Tái Mì Yào*. It's author and exact date of publication are unknown.

Song 歌曰:

一劑分服五錢匕，
五片生薑一棗餌，
枚半附子鎮風虛，
二朮一草君須記 。

Divide one batch into doses of five *qián*-spoons full [each],
Five slices of *shēng jiāng* and one piece of *dà zǎo* for bait,
A piece and a half of *fù zǐ* to settle the wind vacuity,
Six grams of *bái zhú* and three of *gān cǎo*, you must remember this!

Quotation by Yù Jiāyán 喻嘉言云:

（一）此方全不用風藥，但以附子暖其水臟，朮、草暖其土臟。
（二）水土一暖，則濁陰之氣盡趨於下，而頭重苦眩及食不知味之證除矣。

(1) This formula does not use any wind medicinals at all, but only uses *fù zǐ* to warm the water viscus and *bái zhú* and *gān cǎo* to warm the earth viscus.
(2) When water and earth are both warm, the turbid yīn qì all rushes into the lower body. Subsequently, the symptoms of heaviness, bitter pain, dizziness in the head, and not knowing the flavor of food are all eliminated!

崔氏八味丸

Cuī Shì Bā Wèi Wán

Master Cuī's Eight-Ingredient Pills

治腳氣上入少腹不仁 。

A treatment for leg qì ascending and entering the lesser abdomen, causing numbness.

即腎氣丸，見婦人科 。

This is identical with *Shèn Qì Wán*. See [the section on] gynecology.

乾地黃（ 八兩 ）山茱萸 薯蕷（ 各四兩 ）澤瀉 茯苓 牡丹皮（ 各三兩 ）桂枝 附子（ 炮 ）各一兩

gān dì huáng	乾地黃		24g
shān zhū yú	山茱萸		12g
shǔ yù	薯蕷		12g
zé xiè	澤瀉		9g
fú líng	茯苓		9g
mǔ dān pí	牡丹皮		9g
guì zhī	桂枝		3g
fù zǐ	附子	blast-fried	3g

上八味末之，煉蜜和丸梧子大，酒下十五丸，加至二十五丸，日再服 。

Process the eight ingredients above into a powder and combine with refined honey to form pills the size of firmiana seeds.[51] Swallow fifteen pills [per dose] with liquor, increasing the dosage to a maximum of twenty-five pills, two doses per day.

51. A common ancient measurement for medicinal pills, ca. 5-6 mm.

千金越婢加朮湯

Qiān Jīn Yuè Bì Jiā Zhú Tāng

Maid-Servant from Yuè with White Atractylodes from the *Bèi Jí Qiān Jīn Yào Fāng*[52]

歌見水氣病。

For the song, see [the section on] "Water Qì Conditions."

治內極熱，則身體津脫，腠理開，汗大泄，厲風氣，下焦腳弱。

A treatment for extreme heat on the inside that results in desertion of liquids all over the body, open interstices, severe discharge of sweat, pestilence wind qì, and weakness in the lower burner and feet.

麻黃（六兩）石膏（半斤）甘草（二兩）生薑（三兩）白朮（四兩）大棗（十二枚）

má huáng	麻黃	18g
shí gāo	石膏	24g
gān cǎo	甘草	6g
shēng jiāng	生薑	9g
bái zhú	白朮	12g
dà zǎo	大棗	12 pcs

（一）上六味，以水六升，先煮麻黃。（二）去上沫，內諸藥，煮取三升。（三）分溫三服。（四）惡風加附子一枚。

(1) Of the six ingredients above, first simmer the *má huáng* in 1,200ml of water.
(2) Remove the foam from the top, add all the other medicinals, and simmer until reduced to a 600ml
(3) Divide and take heated in three doses.
(4) For aversion to wind, add one piece of *fù zǐ*.

52. See p. 173 below.

Commentary by [Chén] Yuánxī 元犀按:

（一）方中朮、甘、薑、棗，所以維正氣之根，不使陽隨汗出，陰隨熱化也。（二）惡風加附子者，所以預防其亡陽也。

(1) The reason for the presence of *bái zhú, gān cǎo, shēng jiāng,* and *dà zǎo* in this formula is that they safeguard the root of right qì and [thereby] prevent yáng from exiting along with the sweat and prevent yīn from transforming along with the heat.
(2) The reason for adding *fù zǐ* in [patients with] aversion to wind is that you thereby prevent yáng collapse.

血痹虛勞方
Xuè Bì Xū Láo Fāng

Formulas for Blood Impediment and Vacuity Taxation

黄芪桂枝五物湯
Huáng Qí Guì Zhī Wǔ Wù Tāng
Astragalus and Cinnamon Twig Five Substances Decoction

治血痹，陰陽俱微，寸口關上微，尺中小緊，外證身體不仁，如風痹狀。

A treatment for blood impediment with diminution of both yīn and yáng, which manifest with a *cùn kǒu* pulse that is faint on the *guān* position and small and tight in the *chǐ* position,[53] and with the external signs of numbness all over the body and an appearance like wind impediment.

黄芪芍藥桂枝（各三兩）生薑（六兩）大棗（十二枚）

huáng qí	黄芪	9g
sháo yào	芍藥	9g
guì zhī	桂枝	9g
shēng jiāng	生薑	18g
dà zǎo	大棗	12 pcs

上五味，以水六升，煮取二升，溫服七合，日三服。

Simmer the five ingredients above in 1,200ml of water until reduced to 400ml. Take 140ml [per dose] heated, three doses a day.

53. Another possible translation of this line is: "A *cùn kǒu* pulse that is faint above the *guān* position and small and tight in the middle of the *chǐ* position."

Song 歌曰:

血痹如風體不仁，
桂枝三兩芍芪均，
棗枚十二生薑六，
須令陽通效自神。

For blood impediment that looks like wind with generalized numbness,
Nine grams of *guì zhī* and the same amount of *sháo yào* and *huáng qí,*
Twelve pieces of *dà zǎo* and eighteen grams of *shēng jiāng,*
Must cause yáng to flow freely with an efficacy that is naturally divine.

Commentary by [Chén] Yuánxī 元犀按:

（一）內經云: 邪入於陰則為痹。（二）然血中之邪，以陽氣傷而得入，亦必以陽氣通而後出。（三）上節云: 宜針引陽氣，此節而出此方，此以藥代針引之意也。

(1) The *Huáng Dì Nèi Jīng* said: "Evil that enters into yīn results in impediment [patterns]."[54]
(2) The evil in the blood takes advantage of damaged yáng qì to obtain entry and must then also flow along with yáng qì and exit subsequently.
(3) The *Huáng Dì Nèi Jīng* paragraph mentioned above states: "It is appropriate to use the needle to conduct yáng qì." The fact that the present section puts forth this formula here means that it uses medicinals to substitute for the needle in conducting [qì].

Additional Commentary 又按:

（一）此即桂枝湯去甘草之緩，加黃芪之強有力者，於氣分中調其血。（二）更妙倍用生薑以宣發其氣，氣行則血不滯而痹除，此夫倡婦隨之理也。

(1) This formula is in fact *Guì Zhī Tāng* without the moderating effect of *gān cǎo* but with the addition of the force and strength of *huáng qí* to balance the blood via the qì aspect.
(2) Even more ingenious, it doubles the use of *shēng jiāng* to diffuse qì, and when qì moves, blood no longer stagnates and the impediment is eliminated. This is the principle of the husband proposing and the wife following.

54. This quotation is from the *Sù Wèn* 素問 (*Elementary Questions*), chapter 23.

桂枝龍骨牡蠣湯

Guì Zhī Lóng Gǔ Mǔ Lì Tāng

Cinnamon Twig Decoction with Dragon Bone and Oyster Shell Added

（一）治失精家，少腹弦急，陰頭寒，目眩，發落，脈極虛、芤、遲，為清穀、亡血、失精。（二）脈得諸芤動微緊，男子失精，女子夢交，此湯主之。

(1) A treatment for patients suffering from seminal loss that is accompanied by bowstring tension in the lesser abdomen, cold in the tip of the penis, dizzy vision, hair loss, and a pulse that is extremely vacuous, scallion-stalk, and slow, which means clear-grain [diarrhea], blood collapse, or seminal loss.
(2) When you obtain a pulse that is scallion-stalk, stirring, faint, and tight, in men it means seminal loss and in women dreams of intercourse with ghosts. This decoction rules this [condition].

桂枝 芍藥 生薑（各三兩）甘草（二兩）大棗（十二枚）龍骨 牡蠣（各三兩）

guì zhī	桂枝	9g
sháo yào	芍藥	9g
shēng jiāng	生薑	9g
gān cǎo	甘草	6g
dà zǎo	大棗	12 pcs
lóng gǔ	龍骨	9g
mǔ lì	牡蠣	9g

上七味，以水七升，煮取三升，分溫三服。

Simmer the seven ingredients above in 1,400ml of water until reduced to 600ml. Divide and take heated in three doses.

Song 歌曰：

男子失精女夢交，
坎離救治在中爻；
桂枝湯內加龍牡，
三兩相勻要細敲 。

For seminal loss in men and dreams of intercourse with ghosts in women,
To leave the trap and rescue in treatment intertwines in the center.
To *Guì Zhī Tāng* add *lóng gǔ* and *mǔ lì,*
In equal amounts of nine grams each, to strike with care.

Quotation from the *Xiǎo Pǐn Fāng*[55] 小品云：

虛弱浮熱汗出者，除桂加白薇一兩五錢，附子一兩，名曰二加龍骨湯。

For vacuity, weakness, superficial heat, and sweating, eliminate the *guì zhī* and add seven grams of *bái wēi* instead. [With these modifications], the formula is called *Two-Additions Lóng Gǔ Tāng.*

Quotation by Master Xú[56] 徐氏云：

（一）桂枝湯，外證得之能解肌去邪氣，內證得之能補虛調陰陽。
（二）加龍骨、牡蠣者，以失精夢交為神精間病，非此不足以斂其浮越矣。

(1) With *Guì Zhī Tāng,* if the patient has contracted the external signs, you are able to resolve the flesh and get rid of evil qì; if the patient has contracted the internal signs, you are able to supplement vacuity and balance yīn and yáng.
(2) Concerning the addition of *lóng gǔ* and *mǔ lì,* given that seminal loss and dreams of intercourse with ghosts are conditions in the realm of the spirit and essence, if you do not have these [two ingredients], the formula will be insufficient to restrain them from floating astray.

---

55. The *Xiǎo Pǐn Fāng* 小品方 (*Sketched Formulas*) is a collection of formulas predating the *Táng* dynasty that was written in the late fifth century by Chén Yánzhī 陳延之.

56. This is most likely a reference to Xú Língtāi 徐靈胎 (1693-1771), the famous scholar-physician from the *Qīng* period.

Commentary by [Chén] Yuánxī 元犀按:

（一）徐忠可以龍骨、牡蠣斂其浮越四字括之，未免以二味為澀藥，猶有人之見存也。（二）吾於龍之飛潛，見陽之變化莫測；於海之潮汐，見陰之運動不窮。（三）龍骨乃龍之脫換所遺，牡蠣乃海之精英所結，分之為對待之陰陽，合之為各具之陰陽，亦為互根之陰陽，難以一言盡也。（四）其治效無所不包，余亦恐舉一而漏万，惟能讀本經、內經、仲景書者，自知其妙。

(1) Xú Zhōngkě's[57] summary in four characters that *lóng gǔ* and *mǔ lì* are able to "restrain [the spirit and essence] from floating astray" is truly something that anybody can see since the two ingredients are unavoidably astringent medicinals.
(2) I myself see the unfathomable changes of yáng reflected in the flying high and diving low of the dragon, as I see the neverending movement of yīn in the ebb and flow of the ocean.
(3) *Lóng gǔ*[58] is the remains left behind by the dragon when molting, *mǔ lì* is the bound-together quintessence of the ocean. Separately, they are used to deal with yīn and yáng; in combination they are yīn and yáng in mutual completion; they are also yīn and yáng as rooted in each other. It is difficult to fully exhaust this subject in a single word.
(4) In the efficacy of its treatment, there is nothing that it does not embrace. I also fear that I am raising one issue and leaving out a myriad others. If only you can study the *Shén Nóng Běn Cǎo Jīng* and *Huáng Dì Nèi Jīng* and Zhāng Zhòngjǐng's writings, you will know its subtlety on your own.

57. A successful physician who was a disciple of Yù Jiāyán 喻嘉言.

58. The description here of the flight of the dragon is a reference to the first hexagram of the *Yì Jīng* (*Classic of Changes*), lines 1 and 5. Moreover, the reference to the dragon is related to the substance *lóng gǔ* (lit. dragon bones) and the reference to the ocean to the substance *mǔ lì* (oyster shell).

天雄散

Tiān Xióng Sǎn

Tiān Xióng Aconite Powder

天雄（ 三兩 ）白朮（ 八兩 ）桂枝（ 六兩 ）龍骨（ 三兩 ）

tiān xióng	天雄	9g
bái zhú	白朮	24g
guì zhī	桂枝	18g
lóng gǔ	龍骨	9g

上四味，杵為散，酒服半錢匕，日三服，不知，稍增之 。

Process the four ingredients above by pestling into a power and take half a *qián*-spoon with liquor, three doses a day. If you do not notice [any change], increase the dosage bit by bit.

Quotation by Yóu Zàijīng 尤在涇云:

此疑後人所附，為補陽攝陰之用也。

I suspect that this formula has been attached by a later person, for the purpose of supplementing yáng and conserving yīn.

Song 歌曰:

陰精不固本之陽，
龍骨天雄三兩匡，
六兩桂枝八兩朮，
酒調錢匕日三嘗 。

When yīn essence fails to secure yáng at the root,
Nine grams of *lóng gǔ* and *tiān xióng* will correct it.

Eighteen grams of *guì zhī* and twenty-four grams of *bái zhú*,
A *qián*-spoon full mixed into liquor, three tastes a day.

Commentary by [Chén] Yuánxī 元犀按:

（一）此方雖系後人采取，然卻認出春之腳，陽之家，而施以大溫大補大鎮納之劑，可謂有膽有識。（二）方中白朮入脾以納穀，以精生於穀也；桂枝入膀胱以化氣，以精生於氣也；龍骨具龍之性，龍能致水，以海為家，蓋以精歸於腎，猶水歸於海而龍得其安宅也。（三）深得難經所謂損其腎者，益其精之旨。（四）然天雄不得，可以附子代之，斷不可泥於小家天雄主上、附子主下之分。

(1) In spite of the fact that this formula belongs to those inserted by posterity, we can nevertheless recognize that it has its footing in spring and its home in yáng, and is a preparation that applies great warming, great supplementation, and great settling and promotion of absorption. Hence it can be said to have both courage and wisdom.
(2) Within the formula, *bái zhú* enters the spleen to promote the absorption of grain, based on the principle that essence is engendered by grain. *Guì zhī* enters the bladder to promote qì transformation, based on the principle that essence is engendered by qì.
(3) [The formula] deeply grasps the meaning of the saying from the *Nàn Jīng*,[59] "in patients who have injured their kidney, boost the essence."
(4) If *tiān xióng* cannot be obtained, you can substitute *fù zǐ*. You may absolutely not be befuddled by the differentiation of minor masters [in the art of medicine] that *tiān xióng* rules the upper body and *fù zǐ* rules the lower body.

59. *The Classic of Difficulties.*

小建中湯

Xiǎo Jiàn Zhōng Tāng

Minor Center-Strengthening Decoction

見長沙方歌括 。

[For the song], see the *Cháng Shā Fāng Gē Kuò*.

治虛勞，裡急，悸，衄，腹中痛，夢失精，四肢痠疼，手足煩熱，咽乾口燥者主之 。

A treatment for vacuity taxation [that presents with] abdominal urgency, palpitations, nosebleed, pain in the center of the abdomen, seminal loss when dreaming, soreness in the four limbs, vexing heat in the hands and feet, and dry throat and mouth. [This formula] rules it.

桂枝（ 三兩，去皮 ）甘草（ 二兩，炙 ）大棗（ 十二枚 ）芍藥（ 六兩 ）生薑（ 三兩 ）膠飴（ 一升 ）

guì zhī	桂枝	bark removed	9g
gān cǎo	甘草	honey-fried	6g
dà zǎo	大棗		12 pcs
sháo yào	芍藥		18g
shēng jiāng	生薑		9g
jiāo yí	膠飴		200ml

上六味，以水七升，煮取三升，去滓，內膠飴更上微火消解，溫服一升，日三服 。

Simmer the six ingredients above in 1,400ml of water until reduced to 600ml. Remove the dregs, add the *jiāo yí*, and again place on low heat until [the *jiāo yí*] is dispersed. Take 200ml per dose heated, three doses per day.

Quotation by Zhāng Xīnzài 張心在云：

（一）肺損之病，多由五志生火，銷鑠金臟，咳嗽發熱，漸至氣喘，側眠，消瘦羸瘠，虛證交集，咽痛失音而不起矣。（二）壯水之主，以制陽光。（三）王冰成法，於理則通，而多不效，其故何歟？（四）竊嘗觀於爐中之火而得之，炊飯者始用武火，將熟則掩之以灰。（五）飯徐透而不焦黑，則知以灰養火，得火之用而無火之害，斷斷如也。（六）五志之火內燃，溫脾之土以養之，而焰自息，方用小建中湯。（七）虛甚加黄芪，火得所養而不燃，金自清肅；又況飴糖為君，治嗽妙品，且能補土以生金，肺損雖難著手，不患其不可治也。（八）然不獨治肺損，凡五勞七傷，皆可以通治。

(1) Conditions of injury to the lung are mostly caused by the five minds[60] engendering fire, which smelts the viscus of metal. [As a result we see] coughing with heat effusion, gradually leading to panting, sleeping on the side, emaciation and weakness, vacuity signs piling up on top of each other, pain in the pharynx with loss of voice, and inability to get up.
(2) Strengthen the rule of water to restrain the brightness of yáng.
(3) The method created by Wáng Bīng is to establish free flow by means of rectification, and yet it is mostly ineffective. What is the reason for this?
(4) I once observed the fire inside the stove and grasped [the reason]. When cooking rice, we start with a vigorous flame but when the rice is almost done, we cover [the flame] up with the ashes.
(5) The rice is slowly penetrated by this but without being scorched black, hence we know that the ashes are used to nurture the fire. [In this way,] we obtain the use of the fire but avoid the harm done by fire. It is plain and simple like this.
(6) When the fire of the five minds is ignited inside, we warm spleen earth to nurture it, and [as a result] the flames go out on their own. The formula uses *Xiǎo Jiàn Zhōng Tāng* to do just that.
(7) For cases where the vacuity is extreme, add *huáng qí*. The fire will receive nourishment without being inflamed, and metal will naturally return to its function of clearing and eliminating. Furthermore, *yí táng*[61] is the sovereign. It is a wonderful substance for treating cough and is also able to supplement earth and thereby engender metal. Even though injuries of the lung are difficult to put your hands on, do not worry that you are unable to treat them.
(8) [This formula] not only treats injuries of the lung, but all the five taxations and seven damages. All of these can be treated with it.

60. This refers to joy, anger, grief, worry, and fear.

61. I.e., *jiāo yí*.

黄芪建中湯

Huáng Qí Jiàn Zhōng Tāng

Astragalus Center-Strengthening Decoction

治虛勞裡急，諸不足者主之。

A treatment that rules vacuity taxation with abdominal urgency and the various conditions of insufficiency.

即小建中湯加黃耆，一兩五錢。

huáng qí	黄芪		4.5g
guì zhī	桂枝	bark removed	9g
gān cǎo	甘草	honey-fried	6g
dà zǎo	大棗		12 pcs
sháo yào	芍藥		18g
shēng jiāng	生薑		9g
jiāo yí	膠飴		200 ml

（一）即小建中湯加黃芪一兩五錢。（二）氣短胸滿者，加生薑；腹中滿者，去棗加茯苓一兩半；及療肺虛損不足，補氣，加半夏三兩。

(1) This is exactly the same as *Xiǎo Jiàn Zhōng Tāng* [Minor Center-Strengthening Decoction] with the addition of four-and-a-half grams of *huáng qí*.
(2) For shortness of breath and fullness in the chest, add *shēng jiāng*. For fullness in the center of the abdomen, remove the *dà zǎo* and add four-and-a-half grams of *fú líng*. To also cure vacuity detriment and insufficiency in the lung by supplementing qì, add nine grams of *bàn xià*.

Song 歌曰:

小建湯加兩半芪，
諸虛裡急治無遺;
急當甘緩虛當補，
愈信長沙百世師。

Xiǎo Jiàn Zhōng Tāng with the addition of four-and-a-half grams of *huáng qí* [is used]
For all vacuity [conditions] with abdominal urgency, to treat when there is nothing left;
Urgently use sweetness to moderate the vacuity, which you must supplement
For the cure, trust the teacher of a hundred generations from Cháng Shā.

Song for Modifications 加減歌曰:

氣短胸滿生薑好，
三兩相加六兩討;
如逢腹滿脹難消，
加茯兩半除去棗。
及療肺虛損不足，
補氣還須開竅早，
三兩半夏法宜加，
蠲除痰飲為至寶。

For shortness of breath and fullness in the chest, *shēng jiāng* is good,
Nine grams added to a total of eighteen grams can be discussed.
If you come across abdominal fullness, distention, and difficulties with dispersal,
Add four-and-a-half grams of *fú líng* and remove the *dà zǎo*.
To cure vacuity detriment and insufficiency in the lung,
Supplement qì, and you must also open the orifices early,
The method of nine grams of *bàn xià* is a suitable addition.
Abolishing phlegm-rheum is the ultimate treasure.

Commentary by [Chén] Yuánxī 元犀按:

（一）虛勞裡急者，裡虛脈急也；諸不足者，五臟陰精陽氣俱不足也。（二）經云：陰陽俱不足，補陰則陽脫，瀉陽則陰竭，如是者，當調以甘藥。（三）又云：針藥所莫及，調以甘藥，故用小建中湯。（四）君以飴糖、甘草，本稼穡作甘之味，以建立中氣，即內經所謂“精不足者，補之以味”是也。（五）又有桂枝、薑、棗之辛甘，以宣上焦陽氣，即內經所謂”辛甘發散為陽”是也。（六）夫血氣生於中焦，中土虛則木邪肆，故用芍藥之苦泄，於土中瀉木，使土木無忤，而精氣以漸而復，虛勞諸不足者，可以應手而得耳。（七）加黃芪者，以其補虛塞空，貫腠通絡，尤有專長也。

(1) In all cases of vacuity taxation with abdominal urgency, there is vacuity in the interior and an urgent pulse. In all cases of insufficiency, the yīn essence and yáng qì in the five viscera are all insufficient.
(2) The classic states: "Whenever yīn and yáng are both insufficient, supplementation of yīn results in desertion of yáng and draining yáng results in exhaustion of yīn." If conditions are like this, you must balance them by means of sweet medicinals.
(3) It further states: "When needles and medicinals are unable to reach, harmonize with sweet medicinals. For this reason, use *Xiǎo Jiàn Zhōng Tāng*.
(4) With ***yí táng*** and ***gān cǎo*** as sovereigns, the grain crops[62] at the root make the flavor [of this formula] sweet and thereby establish center qì, as said in the *Huáng Dì Nèi Jīng*: "In cases with insufficiency of essence, supplement it with the flavor."[63]
(5) Furthermore, the acrid sweetness of ***guì zhī, shēng jiāng***, and ***dà zǎo*** is used to perfuse yáng qì in the upper burner, as said in the *Huáng Dì Nèi Jīng*: "Acrid and sweet [medicinals], which effuse and dissipate, are yáng."[64]
(6) Now blood and qì are engendered in the center burner. When central earth is vacuous, wood evil runs rampant. Therefore use the bitterness of ***sháo yào*** to discharge, and drain wood from earth in the center. This prevents hostility between earth and wood, and essence and qì thereby gradually recover. In this way, vacuity taxation and all insufficiencies can be addressed effectively.
(7) The addition of ***huáng qí*** has the purpose of supplementing vacuity, plugging up emptiness, and promoting passage through interstices and free flow in the network vessels. This is the special outstanding skill of this formula.

62. I.e., *yí táng* (malt), which is made from grain (i.e. barley).
63. This quotation comes from *Sù Wèn*, chapter 4.
64. This quotation comes from *Sù Wèn*, chapter 74.

八味腎氣丸
Bā Wèi Shèn Qì Wán
Eight Ingredient Kidney Qì Pills[65]

治虛勞腰痛，少腹拘急，小便不利者，此丸主之。

For the treatment of vacuity taxation and lumbar pain with hypertonicity in the lesser abdomen and inhibited urination. These pills rule.

甘地黃（八兩）山藥 山茱萸（各四兩）澤瀉 牡丹皮 茯苓（各三兩）
桂枝 附子（炮）（各一兩）

gān dì huáng	乾地黃		24g
shān yào	山藥		12g
shān zhū yú	山茱萸		12g
zé xiè	澤瀉		9g
mǔ dān pí	牡丹皮		9g
fú líng	茯苓		9g
guì zhī	桂枝		3g
fù zǐ	附子	blast-fried	3g

上八味末之，煉蜜和丸梧子大，酒下十五丸，加至二十五丸，日再服。

Process the eight ingredients above into a powder and combine with refined honey to form pills the size of firmiana seeds. Swallow fifteen pills [per dose] with liquor, increasing the dosage to a maximum of twenty-five pills, two doses per day.

65. This formula is originally found in the volume on gynecology in the *Jīn Guì Yào Lüè*.

薯蕷丸

Shǔ Yù Wán

Dioscorea Pill

治虛勞諸不足，風氣百疾 。

A treatment for vacuity taxation with all forms of insufficiency and the hundred disorders of wind qì.

薯蕷[66](三十分)人參(七分)白朮(六分)茯苓(五分)甘草(二十分)當歸(十分)芍藥(六分)芎藭(六分)乾地黃(十分)麥冬(六分)阿膠(七分)乾薑(三分)大棗(百枚為膏)桔梗(五分)杏仁(六分)桂枝(十分)防風(六分)神曲(十分)柴胡(五分)白蘞(二分)豆黃卷(十分)

shǔ yù	薯蕷		22.5g
rén shēn	人參		5.25g
bái zhú	白朮		4.5g
fú líng	茯苓		3.75g
gān cǎo	甘草		15g
dāng guī	當歸		7.5g
sháo yào	芍藥		4.5g
chuān xiōng	川芎		4.5g
gān dì huáng	乾地黃		7.5g
mài mén dōng	麥門冬		4.5g
ē jiāo	阿膠		5.25g
gān jiāng	乾薑		2.25g
dà zǎo	大棗	processed into a paste	100 pcs
jié gěng	桔梗		3.75g
xìng rén	杏仁		4.5g
guì zhī	桂枝		7.5g

66. *Shŭ Yù* is an alternate name for *shān yào* 山藥.

fáng fēng	防風	4.5g
shén qū	神曲	7.5g
chái hú	柴胡	3.75g
bái liǎn	白蘞	1.5g
dòu huáng juǎn	豆黃卷	7.5g

上二十一味末之，煉蜜和丸如彈子大，空腹酒服一丸，一百丸為劑。

Process the twenty-one ingredients above into a powder and combine with refined honey to form pellet-sized pills. On an empty stomach, take one pill [per dose] with liquor. A hundred pills make up one batch.

Song 歌曰:

三十薯蕷二十草，
三薑二蘞百枚棗，
桔茯柴胡五分勻，
人參阿膠七分討；
更有六分不參差，
芎芍杏防麥朮好，
豆卷地歸曲桂枝，
均宜十分和藥搗；
蜜丸彈大酒服之，
盡一百丸功可造，
風氣百疾並諸虛，
調劑陰陽為至寶。

Twenty-two-and-a-half grams of *shǔ yù*, fifteen of *gān cǎo*,
Two-and-a-quarter of *gān jiāng*, one-and-a-half of *bái liǎn*, and a hundred pieces of *dà zǎo*,
Three-and-three-quarter grams each of *jié gěng*, *fú líng*, and *chái hú*,
Of *rén shēn* and *ē jiāo*, five grams are discussed.
Additionally four-and-a-half grams each with no difference
Of *chuān xiōng*, *sháo yào*, *xìng rén*, *fáng fēng*, *mài mén dōng*, and *bái zhú*;
And of *dòu huáng juǎn*, *dì huáng*, *dāng guī*, *shén qū*, and *guì zhī*
Seven-and-a-half grams each are appropriate. Now combine the medicinals and crush them.
With honey, form into pellet-sized pills and ingest with liquor,
When you have used up all one hundred pills, the effect will be created.
For the hundred disorders of wind qì and all forms of vacuity,
Compounded together, it is the ultimate treasure for yīn and yáng.

Quotation by Wèi Niàntíng[67] 魏念庭曰：

（一）人之元氣在肺，人之元陽在腎，既剝削則難於遽復矣，全賴後天之穀氣資益其生。（二）是營衛非脾胃不能宣通，而氣血非飲食無由平复也。（三）仲景故為虛勞諸不足而兼風氣百疾立此薯蕷丸之法。（四）方中以薯蕷為主，專理脾胃，上損下損，至此可以撑持。（五）以人參、白朮、茯苓、乾薑、豆黄卷、大棗、神曲、甘草助之，除濕益氣，而中土之令得行矣。（六）以當歸、芎藭、芍藥、地黄、麥冬、阿膠養血滋陰。（七）以柴胡、桂枝、防風去邪散熱。（八）以杏仁、桔梗、白蘞下氣開鬱。（九）惟恐虛而有熱之人，滋補之藥上拒不受，故為散其邪熱，開其逆鬱，而氣血平順，補益得納，為至當不易之道也。

(1) A person's original qì lies in the lung; a person's original yáng lies in the kidney. Now in patients suffering from deprivation and whittling away, speedy recovery is difficult because everything relies on the grain qì of later heaven to support and boost its life.
(2) For this reason, construction and defense are unable to perfuse without the spleen and stomach, and qì and blood have no means of calming down and recovering without food and drink.
(3) For this reason, Zhāng Zhòngjǐng established the method of this formula for ***Shǔ Yù Wán*** for vacuity taxation with all forms of insufficiency, complicated by the hundred disorders of wind qì.
(4) In this formula, *shǔ yù* is the ruler, rectifying specifically the spleen and stomach, for detriment in the upper body and detriment in the lower body. By reaching to both [of these places, the effect of the formula] can be sustained.
(5) [The formula] employs *rén shēn, bái zhú, fú líng, gān jiāng, dòu huáng juǎn, dà zǎo, shén qū,* and *gān cǎo* to assist by eliminating dampness and boosting qì, so that the commands of central earth can be carried out.
(6) It employs *dāng guī, chuān xiōng, sháo yào, dì huáng, mài mén dōng* and *ē jiāo* to nourish blood and enrich yīn.
(7) It employs *chái hú, guì zhī,* and *fáng fēng* to remove evil and dissipate heat.
(8) It employs *xìng rén, jié gěng,* and *bái liǎn* to precipitate qì and open depression.
(9) Fearing that in patients suffering from vacuity complicated by the presence of heat the enriching and supplementing medicinals will be rejected above and not received, the formula therefore dissipates the evil heat and opens the counterflow depression, so that qì and blood are calm and smooth, and the supplementing and boosting medicinals can be absorbed. This is the unchanging path of utmost suitability.

67. A physician from the *Qīng* dynasty who composed the *Jīn Guì Yào Lüè Fāng Lùn Běn Yì* 金匱要略方論本義 (*Root Meaning of the Formulas and Essays in the Golden Cabinet*).

酸棗仁湯
Suān Zǎo Rén Tāng
Spiny Jujube Decoction

治虛勞虛煩不得眠。

A treatment for vacuity taxation with vacuity vexation and inability to sleep.

酸棗仁（二升）甘草（一兩）知母（二兩）茯苓（二兩）芎藭（一兩）

suān zǎo rén	酸棗仁	400ml
gān cǎo	甘草	3g
zhī mǔ	知母	6g
fú líng	茯苓	6g
chuān xiōng	川芎	3g

上五味，以水八升，煮酸棗仁得六升，內諸藥煮取三升，分溫三服。

Of the five ingredients above, simmer the *suān zǎo rén* in 1,600ml of water until reduced to 1,200ml. Add all the other medicinals and simmer until reduced to 600ml. Divide and take heated in three doses.

Song 歌曰：

酸棗仁二升先煮湯，
茯知二兩佐之良，
芎甘各一相調劑，
服後恬然足睡鄉。

First simmer 400ml of *suān* **zǎo rén** into a decoction,
Six grams each of *fú líng* and *zhī mǔ* are excellent assistants.
Three grams each of *chuān xiōng* and *gān cǎo,* all compounded together,
After taking it, the patient will be tranquil enough for the land of dreams.

Quotation by Yóu Zàijīng 尤在涇云：

（一）人寤則魂寓於目，寐則魂藏於肝。（二）虛勞之人，肝氣不榮，故以棗仁補斂之。（三）然不眠由於虛煩，必有燥火痰氣之擾，故以知母、甘草清熱滋燥，茯苓、川芎行氣除痰。（四）皆所以求肝之治而宅其魂也。

(1) When people are awake, the *hún* soul resides in the eyes; when they are asleep, it is stored in the liver.
(2) In persons with vacuity taxation, liver qì is not thriving. Therefore use *zǎo rén* to supplement and restrain it.
(3) Now if insomnia is caused by vacuity vexation, it must be related to the harassing presence of dryness, fire, or phlegm qì. Therefore use *zhī mǔ* and *gān cǎo* to clear heat and moisten dryness, and use *fú líng* and *chuān xiōng* to move qì and eliminate dampness.
(4) In all cases the reason we pursue treatment of the liver is that it houses the *hún* soul.

大黃䗪蟲丸
Dà Huáng Zhè Chóng Wán
Rhubarb and Ground Beetle Pill

治五勞虛極羸瘦，腹滿不能飲食，食傷、憂傷、飲傷、房室傷、飢傷、勞傷、經絡營衛氣傷，內有乾血，肌膚甲錯，兩目黯黑，緩中補虛者，此丸主之。

A treatment for the five taxations, extreme vacuity, and marked emaciation, with abdominal fullness and inability to eat and drink, damage from food, damage from anxiety, damage from drinking, damage from sexual intercourse, damage from hunger, damage from taxation, damage to the channels and network vessels and to construction and defense qì, presence of dry blood internally, scaly dry skin, and darkness or blackness in both eyes. By relaxing the center and supplementing vacuity, these pills rule.

大黃（十分，蒸）黃芩（二兩）甘草（三兩）桃仁（一升）杏仁（一升）芍藥（四兩）乾漆（一兩）蚊蟲（一升），乾地黃（十兩）水蛭（百枚）蠐螬（百枚）䗪蟲（半升）

dà huáng	大黃	steamed	7.5g
huáng qín	黃芩		6g
gān cǎo	甘草		9g
táo rén	桃仁		200ml
xìng rén	杏仁		200ml
sháo yào	芍藥		12g
gān qī	乾漆		3g
méng chóng	虻蟲		200ml
gān dì huáng	乾地黃		30g
shuǐ zhì	水蛭		100 pcs
qí cáo	蠐螬		100 pcs
zhè chóng	䗪蟲		100ml

上十二味末之，煉蜜和丸小豆大，酒服五丸，日三服 。

Process the twelve ingredients above into a powder and mix with refined honey to form pills the size of a small bean. Take five pills [per dose] with liquor, three doses a day.

Song 歌曰：

乾血致勞窮源委，
緩中補虛治大旨 。
蠐螬百個䗪半升，
桃杏虻蟲一升止，
一兩乾漆十地黃，
更用大黃十分已，
三甘四芍二黃芩，
五勞要證須用此 。
此方世醫勿惊疑，
起死回生大可恃 。

For dry blood leading to taxation, total exhaustion, and withering at the source,
The main guideline for treatment is to relax the center and supplement vacuity.
A hundred pieces of *qí cáo* and *shuǐ zhì,* 100ml of *zhè chóng,*
Stop at 200ml each of *táo rén, xìng rén,* and *méng chóng,*
Three grams of *gān qī* and thirty of *dì huáng,*
Furthermore use seven-and-a-half grams of *dà huáng* and stop there,
Nine grams of *gān cǎo,* twelve of *sháo yào,* and six of *huáng qín,*
For the key signs of the five taxations, you must use these [ingredients].
This formula, [used by] generations of physicians, do not fear nor doubt!
You can surely trust that it will restore a patient to life even from the point of dying.

Quotation by Yóu Zàijīng 尤在涇曰：

（一）風氣不去，則足以賊正氣而生長不榮，故薯蕷丸為要方。
（二）乾血不去，則足以留新血而滲灌不周，此丸為上劑。

(1) When wind qì fails to leave, it is able to steal right qì and prevent flourishing growth and development. Hence *Shǔ Yù Wán* is the important formula [in such conditions].
(2) When dry blood fails to leave, it is able to cause the retention of new blood, mak-

ing it ooze and pour out rather than circulate. [For this condition], these pills are the supreme preparation.

Personal comment 愚按：

此丸從內經四烏鰂一藘茹丸悟出，但不如四烏鰂一藘茹丸之平易近人也。

These pills come from an understanding of *Sì Wū Zéi Yī Lú Rú Wán*[68] from the *Huáng Dì Nèi Jīng*, but [their action] is not like the smoothness and easy accessibility of *Sì Wū Zéi Yī Lú Rú Wán.*

Quotation by Wáng Jìnsān 王晉三云：

（一）金匱血痹虛勞脈證九條，首條是汗出而風吹之，血凝於膚而為痹，然痹未至於乾血。（二）後六條是諸虛不足而成勞，然勞亦不至於虛极，故治法皆以補虛、和營衛、去風氣為主方。（三）若五勞虛极，痹而內成乾血者，悉皆由傷而血瘀，由血瘀而為乾血也。（四）假如陰之五宮，傷在五味，飲食自倍，則食傷於脾。（五）西方生燥，在臟為肺，在志為憂，憂患不止，則營澀衛除，故憂傷於肺。（六）以酒為漿，以妄為常，女子脫血，醉入房中，則飲傷於肝。（七）嗜欲無窮，精氣弛壞，則房勞傷於腎。（八）谷氣不盈，上焦不行，下脘不通，胃熱陰虧，則飢傷於胃。（九）尊榮人有所勞倦，喘息汗出，其傷在榮，若負重努力人，亦傷於榮，榮氣屬心，故勞傷於心。

(1) The *Jīn Guì Yào Lüè* contains nine sections on the pulses and signs of blood impediment and vacuity taxation. Of these, the first section explains that when a person is sweating and the wind blows on them, blood congeals in the skin and forms impediment. Nevertheless, the impediment does not yet reach the point of dry blood.
(2) The following six sections explain how the various forms of vacuity and insufficiency create taxation, but this taxation still does not reach the point of extreme vacuity. For this reason, the treatment method is always to use ruling formulas that supplement vacuity, harmonize construction and defense, and get rid of wind qì.
(3) In cases where the five taxation and extreme vacuity have lead to impediment and then internally caused the formation of dry blood, this is always a case of damage causing blood stasis and blood stasis in turn causing dry blood.

68. Four of Cuttlefish To One of Madder Pill.

(4) Now if the five palaces of yīn[69] sustain damage from the five flavors because food and drink are doubled, the result is food damage in the spleen.
(5) The western direction engenders dryness. Among the viscera, it is associated with the lung, and among the five minds with anxiety. When anxious worrying is incessant do not stop, construction is astringed and defense is eliminated. The result is anxiety damage in the lung.
(6) Drinking liquor like any [ordinary] beverage, constantly acting frenetically, blood desertion in women, and engaging in sexual intercourse while intoxicated result in drinking damage to the liver.
(7) Having unrestrained [sensuous] cravings that cause essence qì to slacken and spoil result in bedroom taxation damage to the kidney.
(8) When grain qì is not abundant, there is no activity in the upper burner and no flow in the stomach duct in the lower body, and we find heat in the stomach and yīn depletion. The result is hunger damage to the stomach.
(9) When highly respected and honored people experience taxation and fatigue with panting and sweating, their damage is rooted in their honor. [Similarly,] people who have to carry heavy burdens and exert themselves physically also suffer damage in construction, and construction qì belongs to the heart. The result is taxation damage to the heart.

Quotation continued:

（十）諸傷而胃亦居其一者，以五臟皆稟氣於胃，為四時之病變，死生之要會。（十一）胃熱液涸，則五臟絕陰氣之源，而絡痹血乾愈速，故飢傷亦列於臟傷之間。（十二）其第七句是總結諸傷其經絡營衛之氣也。（十三）細繹本文云：腹滿不能食，肌膚甲錯，面目黯黑。明是不能內穀以通流營衛，則營衛凝泣，瘀積之血牢不可破，即有新生之血，亦不得暢茂條達，惟有日漸羸瘦而成內傷乾血勞，其有不死者幾希矣。（十四）仲景乃出佛心仙手，治以 大黃䗪蟲丸。（十五）君以大黃，從胃絡中宣瘀潤燥，佐以黃芩清肺衛，杏仁潤心營，桃仁補肝虛，生地滋腎燥，乾漆性急飛竄，破脾胃關節之瘀血，虻蟲性升，入陽分破血，水蛭性下，入陰分逐瘀，蠐螬去兩脅下之堅血，䗪蟲破堅通絡行陽，卻有神功，故方名標而出之，芍藥、甘草扶脾胃，解藥毒。（十六）緩中補虛者，緩，舒也，綽也，指方中寬舒潤血之品而言也。（十七）故喻嘉言曰：可用瓊玉膏補之，勿以芪、朮補中，失卻寬舒胃氣之義。

(10) In all these damages, the stomach assumes the foremost position, because the five

69. I.e., the heart, liver, spleen, lung, and kidney.

viscera all are endowed with qì by the stomach. It is what determines the transformations of seasonal disease and it is the major meeting point of life and death.
(11) As a result of heat in the stomach and drying up fluids, the five viscera are cut off from the source of yīn qì, and the impediment in the network vessels and dry blood progresses more and more quickly. Therefore hunger damage is also listed among the damages to the viscera.
(12) The seventh sentence [in the *Jīn Guì Yào Lüè*] summarizes the various damages to the qì of the channels and network vessels, construction and defense.
(13) Carefully unravelling the source text, it said "with abdominal fullness and inability to eat and drink, scaly dry skin, and darkness or blackness in both eyes." Elucidating this, if the person is unable to take in grain and thereby free the flow of construction and defense, construction and defense consequently become solidified and weep, static accumulated blood becomes so firm that it is impossible to break it up. Even if there is newly generated blood, it is unable to flow uninhibitedly and profusely and reach out. The patient only becomes more and more emaciated and internally begins suffering from damage from dry blood and taxation. [Among patients like this,] those who do not die are extremely few!
(14) Zhāng Zhòngjǐng truly has extended the heart of a Buddha and the hands of an immortal by treating [this condition] with *Dà Huáng Zhè Chóng Wán.*
(15) The master uses ***dà huáng*** to diffuse stasis and moisten dryness, beginning from inside the stomach network vessels. [This action] is assisted by ***huáng qín,*** which clears lung defense; by ***xìng rén,*** which moistens heart construction; by ***táo rén,*** which supplements liver vacuity; by ***shēng dì huáng,*** which enriches kidney dryness; by ***gān qī,*** which by nature is rash and flies and scurries, breaking up static blood in the spleen and stomach and joints; by ***méng chóng,*** which by nature is upbearing and enters the yáng aspect to break up blood; by ***shuǐ zhì,*** which by nature is precipitating and enters the yīn aspect to expel stasis; by ***qí cáo,*** which removes hardened blood below both rib-sides; by ***zhè chóng,*** which breaks up hardness, frees the flow in the network vessels, and moves yáng. The divine efficacy [of ***zhè chóng***] is the reason why the formula is named after it. The formula includes ***sháo yào*** and ***gān cǎo,*** which prop up the spleen and stomach and resolve the toxicity of the [other] medicinals.
(16) As for "relaxing the center and supplementing vacuity," "relaxing" means smoothing out and widening, and is a reference to those substances in the formula that broaden and smooth out and moisten blood.
(17) Therefore Yù Jiāyán said: "You may use *Qióng Yù Gāo* [Fine Jade Paste] to supplement [this condition], but do not use ***huáng qí*** or ***bái zhú*** to supplement the center. Otherwise you lose the significance of broadening and smoothing out stomach qì.

附方

Fù Fāng

Attached Formulas

千金翼炙甘草湯

Qiān Jīn Yì Zhì Gān Cǎo Tāng

Honey-Fried Licorice Decoction from the *Qiān Jīn Yì Fāng*[70]

歌見長沙方歌括。

For the song, see the *Cháng Shā Fāng Gē Kuò.*

治虛勞不足，汗出而悶，脈結悸，行動如常，不出百日，危急者十一日死。

A treatment for vacuity taxation and insufficiency with sweating and oppression, a bound pulse, and palpitations. [Even though the patient] is active as usual, he or she will not survive for another hundred days, and in cases of extreme danger, will be dead in eleven days.

甘草（四两，炙）桂枝 生薑（各三兩）麥門冬（半升）麻仁（半升）人參 阿膠（各二兩）大棗（三十枚）地黃（一斤）

gān cǎo	甘草	honey-fried	12g
guì zhī	桂枝		9g
shēng jiāng	生薑		9g
mài mén dōng	麥門冬		100ml
má rén	麻仁		100ml
rén shēn	人參		6g
ē jiāo	阿膠		6g

70. 千金翼方 (*Appended Prescriptions Worth a Thousand in Gold*) by Sūn Sīmiǎo 孫思邈.

dà zǎo	大棗	30 pcs
dì huáng	地黄	48g

上九味，以酒七升，水八升，先煮八味，取三升，去滓，內膠消盡，溫服一升，日三服 。

Of the nine ingredients above, first simmer eight of them in 1,400ml of liquor and 1,600ml of water until reduced to a 600ml. Remove the dregs, add the *ē jiāo*, [and mix] until it is completely dissolved. Take 200ml [per dose] heated, three doses per day.

Quotation by Xú[71] 徐云:

（一）此虛勞中潤燥復脈之神方。（二）今人喜用膠、麥等而畏用薑、桂。（三）豈知陰凝燥氣，非陽不能化耶？

> (1) This is a divine formula for moistening dryness and restoring the pulse in the midst of vacuity taxation.
> (2) Nowadays, people like to use [medicinals like] *ē jiāo* and *mài mén dōng* and are afraid of using *shēng jiāng* and *guì zhī*.[72]
> (3) How could they know that [this condition is due to] yīn congealing and dry qì, and is not a case of yáng being unable to transform?

Quotation by Wèi [Niàntíng] 魏云:

仲景用陰陽兩補之法，較後人所制十全、八珍等湯，純美多矣。

Zhāng Zhòngjǐng employs the method of supplementing both yīn and yáng. Compared to formulas like *Shí Quán* [*Dà Bǔ*] *Tāng* or *Bā Zhēn Tāng* that were formulated later, this is much more simple and beautiful.

71. This is most likely a reference to Xú Língtāi 徐靈胎 (1693-1771), the famous scholar-physician from the *Qīng* period.

72. The Chinese here merely says "*jiāng*," which means "ginger" and refers to both dried and fresh ginger. *Ē jiāo* and *mài mén dōng* are mild yīn supplementing medicinals, while *jiāng* and *guì zhī* have a strong yáng-mobilizing and moving effect.

肘後獺肝散

Zhǒu Hòu Tǎ Gān Sǎn

Otter Liver Powder from the *Zhǒu Hòu Bèi Jí Fāng*

治冷勞，又主鬼疰一門相染。

A treatment for cold taxation. [This formula] also rules demonic infixation[73] that has been contracted from another household.

獺肝一具，炙乾末之，水服方寸匕，日三服。

Take one whole liver from an otter and mix-fry until it is dry. Process into a powder. Take one gram in water, three doses per day.

Song 歌曰:

獺肝變化少人知，
一月能生一葉奇；
鬼疰冷勞宜此物，
傳尸蟲蠱是專司。

Of the transformative [power] of liver otter, few people know.
Marvellous how it is able, in one month, to generate one lobe.

73. *Guǐ zhù* 鬼疰: Infixation refers to diseases characterized by infections that become chronically lodged (such as summer infixation, *zhù xià* 疰夏, or worm infixation, *zhù chóng* 疰蟲). It is often used interchangeably with *zhù* 注 (influx) but also carries the connotation of *zhù* 住 (to lodge, stay). In its narrowest and most serious sense as "corpse influx" (*shī zhù* 尸注), it is described in the *Zhū Bìng Yuán Hòu Lùn* 諸病源候論 (*The Origin and Indicators of Disease*) by Cháo Yuánfāng 巢元方 as a dreadful condition caused by externally contracted ghost evil, which leads to increasing suffering from intermittent cold and heat, urinary problems, general severe discomfort, confusion, panting, pain in the abdomen, heart, rib-side, lumbus, and back, and eventually causes the patient's death. Being highly contagious after death, it is likely to be passed on to other members of the family (《諸病源候論》23:2:6). See also Wiseman and Féng, *Practical Dictionary*, p. 300, and《中華醫學大辭典》p. 1087. For a detailed analysis of 疰 by medieval medical writers, see Michel Strickman, *Chinese Magical Medicine*, pp. 23-34.

For demonic infixation and cold taxation, it is suitable to use this ingredient,
It is particularly in charge of [treating] corpse transmission and insect *gŭ*.[74]

Quotation by Wáng Jìnsān 王晉三云:

獺肝散，奇方也。葛稚川治尸疰、鬼疰，仲景治冷癆，皆取用之。

Tă Gān Săn is a marvellous formula. When Gé Zhìchuān[75] treated corpse infixation and demonic infixation, and Zhāng Zhòngjǐng treated cold consumption, both choose this formula in each case.

Commentary 按:

（一）獺肝性溫，能驅陰邪而鎮肝魂，不使魂游於上，而生變動之證。（二）蓋疰者，邪注於臟也。（三）若注於肝，則肝為善變之臟，邪與魂相合，證變便有二十二种，其蟲三日一食，五日一退，變見之證，無非陰象，而獺肝一月生一葉，又有一退葉，是其性亦能消長出入，以殺隱見變幻之蟲。真神品也。

(1) Otter liver is by nature warm and is able to drive out yīn evil and settle the *hún* soul in the liver, preventing the *hún* soul from floating into the upper body and engendering symptoms of transformation and stirring.
(2) Now infixation means that evil has poured into the viscera.
(3) If it has poured into the liver, then the liver, as the viscus that is good at transforming, will mingle with the *hún* soul and you will see the twenty-two types of symptoms of transformation. Its worms will eat once every three days and will retreat once every five days. In terms of the signs that you will see for these transformations, every one of them will be manifestations of yīn. Now the liver of the otter generates one leaf in one month and also has the characteristic of shedding one lobe. This characteristic is also able to [induce] decline and growth, exiting and entering, and thereby kill worms with concealed apparitions and illusionary transformations. It is a truly divine substance.

74. *Gŭ* 蠱: An ancient magical ailment first attested in *Shāng* inscriptions. Originally, it referred to a toxic potion, prepared intentionally by placing several venomous insects in a vessel (as represented by the character) and waiting until all but one of the creatures had died. According to Donald Harper, "demonic bugs or female witchcraft are likely factors in the identity of the ailment" in the *Mă-Wáng-Duī* material (see Donald Harper, *Early Chinese Medical Literature*, pp. 300-301). See also《病源論》25:1 and Paul U. Unschuld, *Medicine in China. A History of Ideas*, pp. 46-50.

75. This is the full name of the author of the *Zhŏu Hòu Bèi Jí Fāng*, who is more commonly known as Gĕ Hóng 葛洪.

卷三
Volume Three

肺痿肺癰咳嗽上氣方
Fèi Wěi Fèi Yōng Ké Sòu Shàng Qì Fāng

Formulas for Lung Wilting, Lung Welling-Abscess, and Cough with Qì Ascent

甘草乾薑湯
Gān Cǎo Gān Jiāng Tāng
Licorice and Dried Ginger Decoction

治肺痿吐涎沫而不咳者，其人不渴，必遺尿，小便數，所以然者，以上虛不能制下故也。此為肺中冷，必眩，多涎唾，以此方溫之。若服湯已渴者，屬消渴。

A treatment for lung wilting with ejection of foamy drool but no cough, in patients who have no thirst but invariably suffer from enuresis and frequent urination. The reason this is so is that the upper body is vacuous and therefore unable to restrain the lower body. This signifies cold inside the lung, which is invariably accompanied by dizziness and an increase in drool and spittle. Warm it by means of this formula. If you see thirst upon taking this formula, this belongs to the category of dispersion-thirst.

甘草（四兩，炙）乾薑（二兩，炮）

gān cǎo	甘草	honey-fried	12g
gān jiāng	乾薑	blast-fried	6g

上㕮咀，以水三升，煮取一升五合，去滓，分溫再服。

Pound the ingredients above and simmer in 600ml of water until reduced to 300ml. Remove the dregs and divide. Take it heated in two doses.

Song 歌曰：

二兩乾薑四炙甘，
薑須炮透旨須探；
傷寒金匱各方中，
止此一方用炮。
肺中津涸方成痿，
氣到津隨得指南 。

Six grams of *gān jiāng* and twelve grams of honey-fried *gān cǎo*,
The *gān jiāng* must be blast-fried and its penetrating aim must be deep.
Among all the formulas of the *Shāng Hán Lùn* and *Jīn Guì Yào Lüè*
It is only this one formula alone that uses it blast-fried.
Only when the fluids inside the lung dry up, wilting forms.
But as the qì arrives, the fluids will follow because they have obtained a guide.

Commentary by Wèi[76] 蔚按：

（一）肺痿皆為熱證，然熱有虛實之不同。（二）實熱宜用寒劑，而此則亡津液而致虛，以虛而生熱。（三）若投以苦寒之劑，非苦從火化而增熱，則寒為熱拒而不納矣。（四）此方妙在以甘草之大甘為主，佐以炮透之乾薑，變其辛溫之性而為苦溫之用，於甘溫除大熱成法中，又參以活法。面面周到，神乎!神乎!

(1) Lung wilting always manifests with heat signs, but the heat can differ depending on whether it is associated with vacuity or repletion.
(2) For repletion heat, it is suitable to use cold preparations. And yet these can result in collapse of the fluids, which leads to vacuity, as a result of which heat is generated.
(3) If you prescribe preparations that are cold and bitter, if the bitterness is not transformed by the fire and increases the heat, the cold [of the medicine] is resisted by the heat and fails to get absorbed!
(4) This formula here is ingenious in that it uses the great sweetness of *gān cǎo* as the ruler, which is assisted by the blast-fried and penetrating *gān jiāng*. [Blast frying the *gān jiāng*] transforms its acrid and warm nature and makes it bitter and warm in effect. Hereby, the formula combines the established method of using the warmth of sweetness to expel great heat with the method of quickening. All-around effective in every aspect, divine indeed, divine indeed!

76. Identity unknown.

射乾麻黃湯
Shè Gān Má Huáng Tāng
Belamcanda and Ephedra Decoction

治咳而上氣，喉中水雞聲者，主之。

A treatment for cough with qì ascent, when there is a sound like a frog in the throat. This formula rules it.

射乾（三兩）麻黃 生薑（各四兩）細辛 紫菀 款冬花（各三兩）大棗（七枚）半夏（半升）五味（半升）

shè gān	射乾	9g
má huáng	麻黃	12g
shēng jiāng	生薑	12g
xì xīn	細辛	9g
zǐ wǎn	紫菀	9g
kuǎn dōng huā	款冬花	9g
dà zǎo	大棗	7 pcs
bàn xià	半夏	100ml
wǔ wèi zǐ	五味子	100ml

上九味，以水一斗二升，先煮麻黃兩沸，去上沫，內諸藥，煮取三升，分溫三服。

Of the nine ingredients above, first simmer the *má huáng* in 2,400ml of water, bringing it a boil twice. Remove the foam on top, add all the other medicinals and simmer until reduced to 600ml. Divide and take heated in three doses.

Song 歌曰:

喉中咳逆水雞聲，
三兩乾辛款菀行，

夏味半升棗七粒，
薑麻四兩破堅城。

For cough in the throat with counterflow and the sound of a frog in the throat,
Nine grams of *shè gān, xì xīn, kuǎn dōng huā,* and *zǐ wǎn* will do,
Of *bàn xià* and *wǔ wèi zǐ* 100ml each, and seven pieces of *dà zǎo,*
Of *shēng jiāng* and *má huáng* twelve grams to break up the wall of hardness.

上方主溫，此方主散。

The previous formula rules by warming. This formula rules by dispersing.

Quotation by Yóu Zàijīng 尤在涇云：

（一）咳而上氣，肺有邪則氣不降而反逆也。（二）肺中寒飲，上入喉間，為呼吸之氣所激，則作聲如水雞。（三）射乾、紫菀、款冬利肺氣；麻黄、細辛、生薑發邪氣；半夏降逆氣，而以大棗安中，五味斂肺，恐劫散之藥并傷及其正氣也。

(1) In cough with qì ascent, there is evil in the lung, which prevents the qì from downbearing and causes it to counterflow in the opposite direction instead.
(2) Cold rheum inside the lung ascends and enters the space of the throat where it irritates inhaled and exhaled qì. As a result, a frog-like sound is produced.
(3) *Shè gān, zǐ wǎn,* and *kuǎn dōng huā* disinhibit lung qì. *Má huáng, xì xīn,* and *shēng jiāng* effuse evil qì. *Bàn xià* downbears counterflow qì. And lastly the formula uses *dà zǎo* to calm the center and *wǔ wèi zǐ* to constrain the lung, because of the fear that the forceful dispersing medicinals also damage the person's right qì.

皂莢丸

Zào Jiá Wán

Gleditsia Fruit Pill

治咳逆上氣，時時吐濁，但坐不得眠者，此丸主之。

A treatment for cough with counterflow qì ascent, constant ejection of turbid [phlegm], and the ability only to sit up but not to lie down. These pills rule.

皂莢（八兩，刮去皮，酥炙）

zào jiá	皂莢	the skin scraped off and honey-fried in ghee	24g

上一味末之，蜜丸梧子大，以棗膏和湯服三丸，日三夜一服。

Process the single ingredient above into a powder and mix with honey to form pills the size of firmiana seeds. Take three pills per dose mixed into *dà zǎo* paste and hot water, three doses per day and one dose at night.

Song 歌曰:

濁痰上氣坐難眠，
癰勢將成壅又堅，
皂莢蜜丸調棗下，
綢繆須在雨之前。

Turbid phlegm with qì ascent and difficulty lying down,
The dynamic of the welling-abscess forms congestion and moreover hardness,
Zào jiá honey pills mixed with *dà zǎo* to get them down,
As a precaution, you must take them [especially] before it rains.

Commentary by Wèi 蔚按:

痰有固而不拔之勢，故用皂莢開其壅閉，滌其污垢，又以棗膏安其胃氣，祛邪中不離養正之法。

Because the phlegm has solidified and the strength to pull it up is lacking, we use *zào jiá* to open the congestion and blockage and to cleanse away its filth, and furthermore use *dà zǎo* paste to calm the person's stomach qì. This is the method for dispelling evil without abandoning [the principle of] nurturing right [qì].

厚朴麻黃湯

Hòu Pò Má Huáng Tāng

Officinal Magnolia Bark and Ephedra Decoction

治咳而脈浮者主之。

A treatment for cough with a floating pulse. This formula rules this condition.

厚朴（五兩）麻黃（四兩）石膏（如雞子大）杏仁（半升）半夏（半升）乾薑細辛（各二兩）小麥（一升）五味（半升）

hòu pò	厚朴	15g
má huáng	麻黃	12g
shí gāo	石膏	1 pc the size of a chicken egg
xìng rén	杏仁	100ml
bàn xià	半夏	100ml
gān jiāng	乾薑	6g
xì xīn	細辛	6g
xiǎo mài	小麥	200ml
wǔ wèi zǐ	五味子	100ml

上九味，以水一斗二升，先煮小麥熟，去滓，內諸藥，煮取三升，溫服一升，日三服。

Of the nine ingredients above, first simmer the *xiǎo mài* in 2,400ml of water until done. Remove the dregs and add all the other medicinals. Simmer until reduced to 600ml, and take 200ml heated, three doses per day.

厚朴麻黄湯

Song 歌曰：

杏仁夏味半升量，
升小麥四麻五朴良，
二兩薑辛膏雞蛋大，
脈浮咳喘此方當 。
一本半夏用至六升，此遵徐注，半夏止用半升。

Of *xìng rén, bàn xià,* and *wǔ wèi zǐ* an amount of 100ml,
200ml of *xiǎo mài,* twelve [grams] of *má huáng* and fifteen of *hòu pò* are excellent.
Six grams of *gān jiāng* and *xì xīn,* and of *shí gāo* a piece the size of a chicken egg,
For a floating pulse with cough and panting, this formula is right.
Other editions use up to 1,200ml of *bàn xià*. Here we follow Xú's[77] notes and stop at using only 100ml of *bàn xià*.

Commentary by [Chén] Yuánxī 元犀按：

（一）咳而脈浮者，內有飲而表有邪也。（二）表邪激動內飲，飲氣上淩，則心肺之陽為之蒙蔽，故用厚朴麻黄湯宣上焦之陽，降逆上之飲。（三）方中厚朴寬胸開蔽；杏仁通泄肺氣，助麻黄解表出邪；乾薑、五味、半夏、細辛化痰滌飲；小麥保護心君。（四）然表邪得辛溫而可散，內飲非質重而難平，故用石膏之質重者，降天氣而行治節，使本飲得就下之性，而無上逆之患也。尤妙先煮小麥，補心養液，領諸藥上行下出，為攘外安內之良圖。（五）可知仲師之方無微不到，學者當細心體認，方得其旨焉。

(1) Cough with a floating pulse means that there is rheum present on the inside and evil in the exterior.
(2) When the evil in the exterior is irritating and stirring the internal rheum and rheum qì encroaches on the upper body, the result is that the yáng of the heart and lung is covered and clouded over. Therefore we use *Hòu Pò Má Huáng Tāng* to perfuse the yáng in the upper burner and to downbear the counterflow ascending rheum.
(3) In the formula, *hòu pò* widens the chest and opens up the cover. *Xìng rén* frees and discharges lung qì and assists *má huáng* in resolving the exterior and expelling the evil. *Gān jiāng, wǔ wèi zǐ, bàn xià,* and *xì xīn* transform phlegm and cleanse away the rheum. *Xiǎo mài* protects the heart as the sovereign.
(4) Nevertheless, even though the evil in the exterior can be dissipated by means of

77. This is most likely a reference to Xú Língtāi 徐靈胎.

acridity and warmth, the internal rheum is not a substance of heavy weight and hence is difficult to calm. Therefore we use the heavy weight of *shí gāo* to downbear heaven's qì and carry out management and regulation, causing the rheum at the root [of the condition] to acquire a downward nature. Thereby, we get rid of the trouble with the counterflow ascent. How ingenious particularly that we first simmer the *xiǎo mài*, which supplements the heart and nourishes liquid and leads all the other medicinals to move in the upper body and to expel from the lower body. This is an excellent plan of resistance on the outside and calming on the inside.

(5) [Based on this] we can know that there is nothing that Teacher Zhòng's[78] formula does not reach. Students must be attentive and use their intuitive knowledge in order to grasp his intention.

78. This is a reference to Zhāng Zhòngjǐng, author of the *Jīn Guì Yào Lüè*.

澤漆湯

Zé Qī Tāng

Sun Spurge Decoction

治咳而脈沉者，此湯主之。

A treatment for cough with a sunken pulse. This decoction rules it.

半夏（半升）澤漆（三升，以東流水五斗，煮取一斗五升）紫參（一本作紫菀[79]）生薑 白前（各五兩）甘草 黃芩 人參 桂枝（各三兩）

bàn xià	半夏		100ml
zé qī	澤漆	simmered in 10 liters of east-flowing water until reduced to 3 liters	600ml
zǐ shēn	紫參		15g
shēng jiāng	生薑		15g
bái qián	白前		15g
gān cǎo	甘草		9g
huáng qín	黃芩		9g
rén shēn	人參		9g
guì zhī	桂枝		9g

上九味，㕮咀，內澤漆湯中煮取五升，溫服五合，至夜盡。

Pound the nine ingredients above and add all to the *zé qī* decoction. Simmer until reduced to 1,000ml. Take 100ml per dose heated. Use it up by nightfall.

Song 歌曰：

五兩紫參薑白前，
三升澤漆法分煎，
桂芩參草同三兩，
半夏半升滌飲專。

79. Another edition uses *zǐ wǎn* 紫菀.

Fifteen grams of *zǐ shēn, shēng jiāng,* and *bái qián,*
600ml of *zé qī*, prepared by simmering it separately,
Of *guì zhī, huáng qín, rén shēn,* and *gān cǎo* nine grams each,
Of *bàn xià* 100ml, a special treatment to sweep away rheum.

Commentary by [Chén] Yuánxī 元犀按：

（一）咳而脈浮者，表有邪也。（二）表邪不解，則乾動內飲而為咳。（三）用厚朴麻黃湯寬胸解表，一鼓而下，則外邪、內飲一并廓清矣。（四）至於咳而脈沉者，里不和也。（五）里氣不和，由於天氣不降，治節不行，而水道不通，致內飲上逆為咳矣。（六）用澤漆湯者，君澤漆，壯腎明，鎮水逆；佐以紫菀、白前，開肺氣，散結氣，以達陽氣；又以半夏、黃芩，分陰陽，安胃氣，以降逆氣，並和裡氣；生薑、桂枝，調營衛，運陽氣，並行飲氣；人參、甘草，奠中土，交陰陽以和之。（七）猶治水者，先修堤岸，以杜其泛濫之患也。（八）先煮澤漆者，取其氣味濃厚，領諸藥入腎，充腎氣，使其吸引有權，則能通府以神其妙用焉。

(1) Cough with a floating pulse means that there is evil present in the exterior.
(2) When the evil in the exterior fails to resolve, the dryness stirs internal rheum and causes the cough.
(3) Using *Hòu Pò Má Huáng Tāng* to widen the chest and resolve the exterior is like conquering the situation with a single strike, because the external evil and internal rheum are both cleared away together.
(4) Now when we talk about cough with a sunken pulse though, it means that the interior is not harmonized.
(5) Qì disharmony in the interior is due to the fact that heaven's qì is fails to downbear, that management and regulation are not being carried out, and that the waterways are not free-flowing, as a result of which internal rheum ascends counterflow and causes cough.
(6) In the application of *Zé Qī Tāng, zé qī* as the sovereign strengthens kidney brightness and settles water counterflow. It is assisted by *zǐ wǎn* and *bái qián,* which open up lung qì and dissipate bound qì in order to outthrust yáng qì. Furthermore, [the formula] uses *bàn xià* and *huáng qín* to separate yīn and yáng and to calm stomach qì, in order to downbear counterflow qì and at the same time harmonize qì in the interior. *Shēng jiāng* and *guì zhī* harmonize construction and defense and transport yáng qì, while at the same time moving rheum qì. *Rén shēn* and *gān cǎo* present the earth at the center and provide an interchange for yīn and yáng, in order to harmonize them.

(7) It is just like managing water: To stop the problem of flooding, you first repair the levees.
(8) The reason we first simmer *zé qī* is that this process removes the thick, dense flavor [and allows it] to lead all the other medicinals to enter the kidney and replenish kidney qì, allowing the patient to inhale with strength. Consequently, we are able to free the palaces[80] and make its ingenious effect divine thereby!

Commentary of teachings received from Lín Lǐfēng[81] 受業林禮豐按：

（一）本方主太陽之裡，太陽底面便是少陰，咳而脈沉者，病在太陽之裡、少陰之表也。（二）蓋太陽主皮毛，邪傷皮毛，必乾於肺，肺傷則不能生水，而少陰之樞逆於下，故立此方。（三）君以澤漆者，以其氣味苦寒，壯腎陰，利水而止咳也，復用白前宣肺氣，黃芩泄肺熱，人參補肺虛，甘草安脾氣，紫菀開結氣，桂枝化膀胱，半夏降逆，生薑滌飲，則肺邪可驅，肺虛可補，腎陰可壯，州都可達矣。（四）煎法先煮澤漆湯，成而後入諸藥者，取其領諸藥以神其妙用也。

(1) This formula rules tàiyáng in the interior and at the bottom of tàiyáng lies shàoyīn. Cough with a sunken pulse means that the disease is located in the interior in taiyang and in the exterior in shàoyīn.
(2) Now tàiyáng rules the skin and body hair, and when evil damages the skin and body hair, it invariably causes dryness in the lung. When the lung is damaged, it is unable to engender water, and the pivot of shàoyīn moves counterflow into the lower body. Therefore this formula is established.
(3) *Zé qī* is the sovereign [of this formula] because its flavor is bitter and cold, and it strengthens kidney yīn and disinhibits water, thereby stopping the cough. The formula additionally employs *bái qián* to diffuse lung qì, *huáng qín* to discharge heat from the lung, *rén shēn* to supplement lung vacuity, *gān cǎo* to calm spleen qì, *zǐ wǎn* to open up bound qì, *guì zhī* for transformation in the urinary bladder, *bàn xià* to downbear counterflow, and *shēng jiāng* to cleanse away rheum. As a result, the evil in the lung can be expelled, the vacuity in the lung can be supplemented, kidney yīn can be strengthened, and all the regions in the body can be outthrust!
(4) The reason the method of decocting is to first simmer *zé qī* into a decoction and when it is done add all the other medicinals, is that it is used to lead all the other medicinals, thereby making the formula's ingenious effect divine!

80. It is unclear whether "palaces" here refers to the yīn bowel organs (i.e. 腑) or to the so-called "mysterious mansions" (玄府), i.e. the sweat pores.

81. Identity of this person is unknown.

麥門冬湯
Mài Mén Dōng Tāng
Ophiopogon Decoction

治火逆上氣，咽喉不利，止逆下氣者，此湯主之。

A treatment for fire counterflow and qì ascent, with inhibition in the throat. To stop counterflow and precipitate qì, this decoction rules.

麥門冬（七升）半夏（一升）人參甘草（各二兩）粳米（三合）大棗（十二枚）

mài mén dōng	麥門冬	1,400ml
bàn xià	半夏	200ml
rén shēn	人參	6g
gān cǎo	甘草	6g
jīng mǐ	粳米	60ml
dà zǎo	大棗	12 pcs

上六味，以水一斗二升，煮取六升，溫服一升，日三夜一服。

Simmer the six ingredients above in 2,400ml of water until reduced to 1,200ml. Take 200ml per dose heated, three doses a day and one dose at night.

Song 歌曰：

火逆原來氣上衝，
一升半夏七升冬，
參甘二兩粳三合，
棗十二枚是正宗。

Fire counterflow originally comes from qì surging into the upper body.
200ml of *bàn xià* and 1,400ml of *mài mén dōng*,

Of *rén shēn* and *gān cǎo* six grams, and 60ml of *jīng mǐ*,
Of *dà zǎo* twelve pieces, this is the correct tradition.

Quotation by Yù Jiāyán 喻嘉言云：

於大建中氣、大生津液隊中，增入半夏之辛溫一味，其利咽下氣，非半夏之功，善用半夏之功，擅古今未有之奇矣!

Among the troop of [medicinals] that strongly establish center qì and strongly engender liquids, there is only a single ingredient added that is acrid and warm, namely *bàn xià*. [The formula's] action of disinhibiting the throat and precipitating qì does not [match the normally intended] effect of *bàn xià*. The skill of employing the effect of *bàn xià* is so rare as to be superior to anything that exists in the past and present!

葶藶大棗瀉肺湯

Tíng Lì Dà Zǎo Xiè Fèi Tāng

Lepidium/Descurainiae and Jujube Lung-Draining Decoction

治肺癰，喘不得臥者，主之。

A treatment for welling-abscesses in the lung with panting and inability to lie down. [This formula] rules it.

葶藶（熬令黃色，搗丸如雞子大）大棗（十二枚）

tíng lì	葶藶	boiled in water until it has turned yellow, and crushed	1 pellet the size of a chicken egg
dà zǎo	大棗		12 pcs

上先以水三升煮棗，取二升，去棗，內葶藶，煮取一升，頓服。

Of the ingredients above, first simmer the *dà zǎo* in 600ml of water until reduced to 400ml. Take out the *dà zǎo*, add the *tíng lì*, and simmer until reduced to 200ml. Drink it down in a single gulp.

Song 歌曰:

喘而不臥肺癰成，
口燥口中關關乾燥胸疼中隱隱痛數實呈；
肺痿數而虛，肺癰脈數而實；
葶藶一丸十二棗，
雄軍直入奪初萌。

Panting and inability to sleep [means that] a lung welling-abscess is forming.
Dry mouth (feeling of dryness in the mouth), chest pain (dull pain in the center), and a rapid replete pulse will manifest.

Lung wilting manifests with a rapid and vacuous pulse, and lung welling abscess with a rapid and replete pulse.

One pellet of *tíng lì* and twelve pieces of *dà zǎo*,
A mighty army that goes right in to snatch up the first sprout.

Quotation by Yóu Zàijīng 尤在涇云:

葶藶苦寒，入肺泄氣閉，加大棗甘溫以和藥力，與皂莢丸之飲以棗膏同法。

Tíng lì is bitter and cold and enters the lung to discharge qì blockage. The addition of *dà zǎo*, which is sweet and warm, is used to harmonize the strength of the medicine. This is the same method that we find in the use of *dà zǎo* paste when drinking down *Zào Jiá Wán*.

桔梗湯
Jié Gěng Tāng
Platycodon Decoction

治肺癰咳而胸滿，振寒脈數，咽乾不渴，時出濁唾腥臭，久久吐膿如米粥者，此湯主之。

A treatment for lung welling-abscess with cough and fullness in the chest, shivering with cold and a rapid pulse, dryness in the throat but without thirst, from time to time expulsion of turbid spittle that smells fishy or foul, and when the condition persists for a very long time, ejection of pus that resembles rice gruel. This decoction governs it.

桔梗（一兩）甘草（二兩）

jié gěng	桔梗	3g
gān cǎo	甘草	6g

上以水三升，煮取一升，分溫再服，則吐膿血也。

Simmer the ingredients above in 600ml of water until reduced to 200ml. Divide and take heated in two doses. [Ingesting this medicine] will result in vomiting of pus and blood.

Song 歌曰：

膿如米粥肺須清，
毒潰難支，藥要輕；
甘草二兮桔一兩，
土金合化得生生。

When there is pus like rice gruel, the lung must be cleared,
Since bursting toxins are difficult to support, the medicine must be light.
Six grams of *gān cǎo* and three of *jié gěng*,
In combination, earth and metal transform and are able to engender life!

Commentary by [Chén] Yuánxī 元犀按:

（一）肺癰尚未成膿，用葶藶瀉之。（二）今已潰後，用此湯排膿解毒，宜緩治，不可峻攻也。（三）余解見長沙方歌括。

(1) Before a welling-abscess in the lung has formed pus, you use *tíng lì* to drain it.
(2) The present [line describes a condition where the abscess] has already burst open, in which case we use this decoction to expel pus and resolve toxin. You should treat in moderation and may not attack fiercely.
(3) For my explanation, see the *Cháng Shā Fāng Gē Kuò*.

越婢加半夏湯

Yuè Bì Jiā Bàn Xià Tāng[82]

Maid-Servant from Yuè with Pinellia Added

治咳而上氣，此為肺脹，其人喘，目如脫狀，脈浮大者，此湯主之。

A treatment for cough with qì ascent, which means lung distention. A patient [with this condition presents with] panting, an appearance as if the eyes were about to fall out, and a pulse that is floating and large. For such cases, this decoction rules.

麻黄（六兩）石膏（半斤）生薑（三兩）大棗（十二枚）甘草（二兩）半夏（半升）

má huáng	麻黄	18g
shí gāo	石膏	24g
shēng jiāng	生薑	9g
dà zǎo	大棗	12 pcs
gān cǎo	甘草	6g
bàn xià	半夏	100ml

上六味，以水六升，先煮麻黄，去上沫，內諸藥，煮取三升，分溫三服。

Of the above six ingredients, first simmer the *má huáng* in 1,200ml of water. Remove the foam from the top, add all the other medicinals, and simmer until reduced to 600ml. Divide and take heated in three doses.

82. In Wiseman terminology, the group of formulas with "*yuè bì*" in the name are translated as "Spleen-Effusing ... Decoctions" but given the much stronger connection to the lung here, this interpretation strikes me as less likely than the more immediate translation as "Maid-Servant from Yuè" (name of an ancient Chinese state).

Song 歌曰：

風水多兮氣亦多，
水風相搏浪滔滔；
全憑越婢平風水，
加夏半升奠巨波。

Excessive wind and water means that qì is also excessive.
When water and wind struggle with each other, waves become torrential.
Everything depends on *Yuè Bì Tāng* to calm the wind and water,
With the addition of 100ml of *bàn xià* to settle giant waves.

Commentary by [Chén] Yuánxī 元犀按：

（一）此肺脹，原風水相搏，熱氣奔騰，上蒸華蓋，走入空竅，故咳而上氣喘，目如脫狀證。（二）脈浮大者，風為陽邪，鼓蕩於其間故也。（三）方用麻黃、生薑直攻外邪；石膏以清內熱；甘草、大棗可補中氣。（四）加半夏以開其閉塞之路，俾肺竅中之痰涎淨盡，終無肺癰之患也。

(1) In this type of distention in the lung, originally wind and water were struggling with each other and heat qì surged roaring upward. Steaming up into the florid canopy,[83] it then ran into the orifices, causing the signs of cough, qì ascent panting, and an appearance as if the eyes are about to fall out.
(2) The pulse is floating and large because wind is a yáng evil and is agitating in the empty spaces.
(3) The formula uses *má huáng* and *shēng jiāng* to directly attack evil on the outside. It uses *shí gāo* to clear heat on the inside. And it uses *gān cǎo* and *dà zǎo* to supplement center qì.
(4) *Bàn xià* is added to open the blocked paths and to completely clean out the phlegm-drool inside the orifices of the lung so that ultimately there will be no more trouble with the lung welling-abscess.

83. I.e. the lung.

小青龍加石膏湯

Xiǎo Qīng Lóng Jiā Shí Gāo Tāng

Minor Green-Blue Dragon Decoction with Gypsum Added

治肺脹，咳而上氣，煩躁而喘，脈浮者，心下有水，此湯主之。

A treatment for distention in the lung with cough and qì ascent, vexation, agitation, and panting, and a floating pulse, which indicates the presence of water below the heart. This decoction rules it.

小青龍方見傷寒論。再加石膏三兩，即此方也。

For the formula for *Xiǎo Qīng Lóng Tāng*, see the *Shāng Hán Lùn*. If you add an additional nine grams of *shí gāo*, you get the present formula.[84]

麻黃芍藥桂枝細辛甘草乾薑（各三兩）五味子半夏（各半升）石膏（二兩）

má huáng	麻黃	knots removed	9g
sháo yào	芍藥		9g
guì zhī	桂枝		9g
xì xīn	細辛		9g
gān cǎo	甘草	honey-fried	9g
gān jiāng	乾薑		9g
wǔ wèi zǐ	五味子		100ml
bàn xià	半夏		100ml
shí gāo	石膏		6g

（一）上九味，以水一斗，先煮麻黃，減二升。（二）去上沫，內諸藥，煮取三升，去滓，溫服一升。（三）強人服一升，羸者減之。日三服，小儿服四合。

84. The formula has been added to the text for the reader's convenience. The addition of *shí gāo* to *Xiǎo Qīng Lóng Tāng* has a precedent in *Dà Qīng Lóng Tāng*, which also includes *shí gāo*. See the commentary below.

(1) Of the nine ingredients above, first simmer the ***má huáng*** in 2,000ml of water until reduced by 400ml.
(2) Remove the foam from the top, add all the other medicinals, and simmer until reduced to 600ml. Remove the dregs, [divide into two doses,] and take 200ml per dose heated.
(3) For strong patients, take 200ml per dose. For emaciated patients, reduce this amount. Take three doses per day. For young children, take 80ml per dose.

Song 歌曰:

小龍分兩照原方，
二兩膏加仔細詳，
水飲得溫方可散，
欲除煩躁藉辛涼。

[Prepare] *Xiǎo Qīng Lóng Tāng* and divide into two doses, according to the original formula.
With the addition of six grams of ***shí gāo***, be careful and attentive.
Only by being exposed to warmth can water-rheum then be dissipated.
If you want to eliminate vexation and agitation, make use of acrid and cool [substances].

Quotation by Yóu Zàijīng 尤在涇云:

（一）此亦內邪外飲相搏之證，但兼煩躁，則挾有熱邪。（二）特加石膏，即大青龍例也。（三）然心下有水，非溫藥不得開而去之，故不用越婢加半夏，而用小青龍加石膏。（四）寒溫並進，水熱俱捐，於法為尤密矣。

(1) This line also describes signs of internal evil and external rheum struggling with each other, but when these are combined with vexation and agitation, it means that the condition is complicated by heat evil.
(2) [In this case,] specifically add ***shí gāo***, which is then an example of *Dà Qīng Lóng Tāng*.
(3) Now, since there is water present below the heart, if you do not include warm medicinals, you will not be able to open up and remove it. Therefore we do not use *Yuè Bì Jiā Bàn Xià Tāng* but instead use *Xiǎo Qīng Lóng Jiā Shí Gāo Tāng*.
(4) Introducing both warmth and cold so that water and heat are both reduced, this method is a very special secret!

Quotation by Wèi Niàntíng 魏念庭云：

（一）師為肺冷而乾燥將痿者，立甘草乾薑湯一方；為肺熱而枯焦將致痿者，立麥門冬湯一方，皆預治肺痿之法也。（二）師為有表邪而肺鬱，恐成痿與癰者，立射乾湯一法；為無外邪而氣上逆者，恐其成癰，立皂莢丸一法；為有外邪而預理其肺者，立厚朴麻黃湯一法；有外邪而復有內熱者，立澤漆湯法，皆預治肺氣，不令成痿癰之意也。（三）又為有外邪而肺脹急，立越婢加半夏湯一法；有外邪而復有內熱，肺脹煩躁者，立小青龍加石膏一法，亦皆預治肺氣，不令成癰痿之意也。（四）主治者果能明此，選擇比屬而用之，又何大患之可成乎？（五）及肺癰已成，用大棗葶藶瀉肺湯；久久吐膿如米粥，用桔梗湯。（六）不以病之不可為而棄之，益見濟人無已之苦心也。

(1) For cases of cold in the lung with dryness about to turn into wilting, the master[85] has established the formula of *Gān Cǎo Gān Jiāng Tāng*. For heat in the lung with parching that is about to turn into wilting, he established the formula of *Mài Mén Dōng Tāng*. Both of these are methods of preventatively treating lung wilting.

(2) For lung depression as the result of evil in the exterior, fearing that it will turn into wilting and welling-abscess, he established the method of *Shè Gān Tāng*. For cases of qì counterflow ascent with no evil present on the outside, fearing that it will turn into welling-abscess, he established the method of *Zào Jiá Wán*. For cases where there is evil present on the outside and you want to preventatively rectify the lung, he established the method of *Hòu Pò Má Huáng Tāng*. For cases where there is evil present on the outside and furthermore there is heat inside, he established the method of *Zé Qī Tāng*. All of these have the intention of preventatively treating lung qì to prevent the formation of wilting or welling-abscess.

(3) Furthermore, for the presence of external evil with distention and tension in the lung, he has established the method of *Yuè Bì Jiā Bàn Xià Tāng*. For the presence of external evil and moreover internal heat with distention in the lung and vexation and agitation, he has established the method of *Xiǎo Qīng Lóng Jiā Shí Gāo Tāng*. Both of these also have the intention of preventatively treating lung qì to prevent the formation of welling-abscess and wilting.

(4) If you can clearly understand the main indications and apply the formula based on a selection by comparison, then what major trouble could possibly appear?

(5) Now if a welling-abscess has already formed in the lung, use *Dà Zǎo Tíng Lì Xiè Fèi Tāng*. If the condition has persisted for a very long time and the patient presents with ejection of pus that resembles rice gruel, use *Jié Gěng Tāng*.

(6) Not to abandon [patients] because the disease cannot be accounted for all the more manifests the excruciating effort of selflessly rescuing others.

85. I.e., Zhāng Zhòngjǐng.

附方
Fù Fāng
Attached Formulas

外台炙甘草湯
Wài Tái Zhì Gān Cǎo Tāng
Honey-Fried Licorice Decoction from the *Wài Tái Mì Yào*

方歌見長沙方歌括 。

For the formula see the *Cháng Shā Fāng Gē Kuò.*

治肺痿涎唾多，心中溫溫液液者 。

A treatment for lung wilting with excessive drool and spittle, with a feeling inside the heart as if overflowing and about to vomit.

Commentary by [Chén] Yuánxī 元犀按:

（一）肺痿涎唾多，心中溫溫液液者，心陰不足也。（二）心陰不足則心陽上熾，勢必克金而成肺痿。（三）方用炙甘草湯生津潤燥，養陰維陽，使陰復而陽不浮，則清肅之令自行於肺矣。（四）余義見傷寒論，不再贅。

(1) "Lung wilting with excessive drool and spittle, with a feeling inside the heart as if overflowing and about to vomit" means insufficiency of heart yīn.
(2) When heart yīn is insufficient, heart yáng blazes upward and its force invariably overcomes metal, causing lung wilting.
(3) The formula uses *Zhì Gān Cǎo Tāng* to engender fluids and moisten dryness, and to nourish yīn and safeguard yáng, causing yīn to return and preventing yáng from floating up. As a result, the command of clearing and eliminating is naturally carried out by the lung.
(4) For my explanation of its meaning, see the *Shāng Hán Lùn*. It is superfluous to repeat it here.

千金甘草湯

Qiān Jīn Gān Cǎo Tāng

Licorice Decoction from the *Bèi Jí Qiān Jīn Yào Fāng*

歌解見長沙方歌括 。

For the song and explanation, see the *Cháng Shā Fāng Gē Kuò.*

gān cǎo　甘草

一味，以水三斗，煮減半，溫分三服 。

Simmer the single ingredient in six liters of water until reduced by half. Take heated, divided into three doses.

千金生薑甘草湯

Qiān Jīn Shēng Jiāng Gān Cǎo Tāng

Fresh Ginger and Licorice Decoction from the *Bèi Jí Qiān Jīn Yào Fāng*

治肺痿咳唾涎沫不止，咽燥而渴 。

A treatment for lung wilting with cough, incessant drooling of foamy spittle, dry throat, and thirst.

生薑（ 五兩 ）人參（ 三兩 ）甘草（ 四兩 ）大棗（ 十五枚 ）

shēng jiāng	生薑	15g
rén shēn	人參	9g
gān cǎo	甘草	12g
dà zǎo	大棗	15 pcs

上四味，以水七升，煮三升，分溫三服 。

Simmer the four ingredients above in 1,400ml of water until reduced to a 600ml. Divide and take heated in three doses.

Song 歌曰:

肺痿唾涎咽燥殃，
甘須四兩五生薑，
棗枚十五參三兩，
補土生津潤肺腸 。

Lung wilting with drooling of spittle and dry throat spells disaster.
Of *gān cǎo* you must use twelve grams, and of *shēng jiāng* fifteen,
Fifteen pieces of *dà zǎo* and nine grams of *rén shēn,*
To supplement earth, engender the fluids, and moisten the lung and intestines.

Commentary by [Chén] Yuánxī 元犀按:

（一）中者，土也。土能生金，金之母，即資生之源也。（二）夫肺痿咳唾涎沫不止，咽燥而渴者，是中土虛，水氣逆，阻其正津不能上滋也。（三）方用生薑甘草湯者，君生薑破陰行陽，蒸津液上滋；佐以人參，入太陰，振脾中之陽，育肺中之陰；又以棗、草助之，為資生之始，令土旺則生金制水矣。

(1) The middle is earth. Earth is able to engender metal and as the mother of metal hence the source of promoting life.

(2) Now lung wilting with cough and incessant drooling of foamy spittle, dry throat, and thirst means vacuity in center earth. Water qì moves counterflow and obstructs the correct flow of liquid so that it is unable to enrich the upper body.

(3) The reason we use the formula *Shēng Jiāng Gān Cǎo Tāng* is that the sovereign *shēng jiāng* breaks up yīn and moves yáng, steams the fluids and enriches the upper body. It is assisted by *rén shēn,* which enters tàiyīn to arouse yáng inside the spleen and foster yīn inside the lung. In addition, with the assistance of *dà zǎo* and *gān cǎo,* [this formula] is the beginning of promoting life, causing earth to prosper so that it can engender metal and restrain water!

千金桂枝去芍藥加皂莢湯
Qiān Jīn Guì Zhī Qù Sháo Yào Jiā Zào Jiá Tāng
Cinnamon Twig Decoction with Peony Removed and Gleditsia Fruit Added
from the *Bèi Jí Qiān Jīn Yào Fāng*

治肺痿吐涎沫。

A treatment for lung wilting with vomiting of drool and spittle.

桂枝生薑（各三兩）甘草（三兩）大棗（十二枚）皂莢（一枚，去皮子，炙焦）

guì zhī	桂枝		9g
shēng jiāng	生薑		9g
gān cǎo	甘草		9g
dà zǎo	大棗		12 pcs
zào jiá	皂莢	skin and seeds removed and honey-fried until scorched	1 pc

上五味，以水七升，微火煮取三升，分溫三服。

Simmer the five ingredients above in 1,400ml of water over gentle heat until reduced to 600ml, divide and take heated in three doses.

Song 歌曰：

桂枝去芍本消陰，
痰飲挾邪迫肺金；
一個皂驅黏膩濁，
桂枝運氣是良箴。

Guì Zhī Tāng minus *sháo yào* at its root disperses yīn,
When phlegm-rheum that is complicated by evil distresses lung-metal.

One piece of *zào jiá* drives out sticky and slimy turbidity,
While *guì zhī* moving qì is an excellent warning.

Commentary by [Chén] Yuánxī 元犀按:

（一）非辛溫之品，不能行陽運氣；非甘潤之品，不能補土生津。（二）君以薑、桂之辛溫，行陽消陰；佐以大棗、甘草之甘潤，補陰生液。（三）若夫開壅塞，滌污垢，以淨其涎沫者，則皂莢尤有專長耳。

(1) Without acrid and warm substances, we are unable to move yáng and transport qì. Without sweet and moistening substances, we are unable to supplement earth and engender fluids.
(2) The acridity and warmth of the sovereigns *shēng jiāng* and *guì zhī* move yáng and disperse yīn. They are assisted by the sweet moistening of *dà zǎo* and *gān cǎo,* to supplement yīn and engender liquid.
(3) If we want to open up the blockage and congestion and wash away the filth, thereby cleaning the foamy drool, *zào jiá* in particular has a special ability to do so.

外台桔梗白散

Wài Tái Jié Gěng Bái Sǎn

Platycodon White Powder from the *Wài Tái Mì Yào*

歌解見長沙方歌括。

For the song, see the *Cháng Shā Fāng Gē Kuò.*

治咳而胸滿，振寒脈數，咽乾不渴，時出濁唾腥臭。久久吐膿如米粥者，為肺癰。

A treatment for cough with fullness in the chest, shivering with cold and a rapid pulse, dry throat but no thirst, and from time to time expulsion of turbid drool that smells fishy or foul. If this condition persists for a very long time and you see ejection of pus that resembles rice gruel, it means welling-abscess in the lung.

桔梗 貝母（各三分）巴豆（一分，去皮，熬，研如霜）

jié gěng	桔梗		2.25g
bèi mǔ	貝母		2.25g
bā dòu	巴豆	skin removed, boiled in water, and ground into a frostlike powder	0.75g

（一）上三味為散，強人飲服半錢匕，羸者減之。（二）病有膈上者吐膿，有膈下者瀉出。（三）若下多不止，飲冷水一杯則定。

(1) Process the three ingredients above into a powder. For strong patients, take half a *qián*-spoon full per dose; for emaciated patients, reduce the amount.
(2) If the disease is located above the diaphragm, there will be ejection of pus. If it is located below the diaphragm, there will be diarrhea.
(3) If there is excessive precipitation that does not stop, drink one cup of cold water to settle it.

千金葦莖湯

Qiān Jīn Wěi Jīng Tāng

Phragmites Stem Decoction from the *Bèi Jí Qiān Jīn Yào Fāng*

治咳有微熱，煩滿，胸中甲錯，是為肺癰。

A treatment for cough with mild heat, vexation and fullness, and scaly dry skin in the center of the chest. This indicates a welling-abscess in the lung.

葦莖（二升）薏苡仁（半升）桃仁（五十粒）栝瓣（半升）

wěi jīng	葦莖	400ml
yì yǐ rén	薏苡仁	100ml
táo rén	桃仁	50 pcs
guā bàn	栝瓣	100ml

上四味，以水一斗，先煮葦莖得五升，去滓，內諸藥煮取二升，服一升，再服，當吐如膿。

Of the four ingredients above, first simmer the *wěi jīng* in 2,000ml of water until reduced to 1,000ml. Remove the dregs, add all the other ingredients, and simmer again until reduced to 400ml. Take 200ml per dose. Two doses should induce ejection of a pus-like substance.

Song 歌曰：

胸中甲錯肺癰成，
煩滿咳痰數實呈；
苡瓣半升桃五十，
方中先煮二升莖。

Dry scaly skin in the center of the chest means that a welling-abscess is forming in the lung. It presents with vexation, fullness, cough with phlegm, and a rapid replete pulse.

100ml of *yì yǐ rén* and *guā bàn*, and fifty pieces of *táo rén*,
In the formula, first simmer the 400ml of *wěi jīng*.

Commentary by [Chén] Yuánxī 元犀按:

（一）此方以濕熱為主。（二）咳有微熱、煩滿、胸中甲錯者，是濕熱之邪結在肺也。（三）肺既結，則阻其氣血不行而為痛矣。（四）方用葦莖解氣分之熱結；桃仁泄血分之熱結；薏苡利濕，清結熱之源；栝瓣排瘀，開結熱之路。（五）方下注云：再服當吐如膿者，指藥力行肺癰潰矣。

(1) This formula takes damp heat as its main indication.
(2) Cough with mild heat, vexation and fullness, and scaly dry skin in the center of the chest means that the evil of damp heat is binding in the lung.
(3) When there is binding in the lung, the result is obstruction of its qì and blood, failure to flow, and therefore pain!
(4) The formula uses *wěi jīng* to resolve the heat bind in the qì aspect; *táo rén* to discharge the heat bind from the blood aspect; *yì yǐ rén* to disinhibit dampness and clear the source of the bound heat; and *guā bàn* to expel stasis and open up the pathways for the bound heat.
(5) The note below the formula that states, "two doses should induce ejection of a pus-like substance," indicates that the force of the medicine is acting on the lung and the welling-abscess has erupted!

葶藶大棗瀉肺湯

Tíng Lì Dà Zǎo Xiè Fèi Tāng

Lepidium/Descurainiae and Jujube Lung-Draining Decoction

治肺癰胸滿脹，一身面目浮腫，鼻塞清涕出，不聞香臭酸辛，咳逆上氣，喘鳴迫塞，此湯主之。

A treatment for welling-abscess in the lung with fullness and distention in the chest, puffy swelling all over the body and in the face and eyes, congestion in the nose with discharge of clear snivel, inability to smell fragrant or foul smells or [taste] sour or acrid substances, cough with counterflow ascent of qì, and raspy panting with distress and congestion. This decoction rules it.

葶藶（熬令黃色，搗丸如雞子大）大棗（十二枚）

tíng lì	葶藶	boiled in water until it has turned yellow, crushed.	A pill the size of a chicken's egg
dà zǎo	大棗		12 pcs

上先以水三升，煮棗取二升，去棗，內葶藶，煮取一升，頓服。

Of the above ingredients, first simmer the *dà zǎo* in 600ml of water until reduced to 400ml. Remove the *dà zǎo*, add the *tíng lì*, and simmer until reduced to 200ml. Take it by drinking it down in a single gulp.

三日一劑，可至三四劑，此先服小青龍湯一劑乃進。

Take one preparation every three days. You can take up to three or four preparations. If you first take one preparation of *Xiǎo Qīng Lóng Tāng*, it will be able to enter [the body].

奔豚方
Bēn Tún Fāng

Formulas for Running Piglet

奔豚湯
Bēn Tún Tāng
Running Piglet Decoction

治奔豚氣上衝胸，腹痛，往來寒熱者，主之 。

A treatment for running piglet with qì surging up into the chest, abdominal pain and alternating cold and heat. [This formula] rules it.

甘草 當歸 芎藭 黄芩 芍藥（ 各二兩 ）半夏 生薑（ 各四兩 ）生葛（ 五兩 ）甘李根 白皮（ 一升 ）

gān cǎo	甘草	6g
dāng guī	當歸	6g
chuān xiōng	川芎	6g
huáng qín	黄芩	6g
sháo yào	芍藥	6g
bàn xià	半夏	12g
shēng jiāng	生薑	12g
shēng gé gēn	生葛根	15g
gān lǐ gēn bái pí	甘李根 白皮	200ml

上九味，以水二斗，煮取五升，溫服一升，日三夜一服 。

Simmer the nine ingredients above in 4,000ml of water until reduced to 1,000ml. Take 200ml per dose heated, three times a day and once at night.

Song 歌曰：

氣衝腹痛號奔豚，
四兩夏薑五兩葛根，
歸芍芎芩甘二兩，
李皮須到一升論 。

Qì surging with abdominal pain is called running piglet.
Twelve grams of *bàn xià* and *gān jiāng* and fifteen grams of *gé gēn,*
Six grams each of *dāng guī, sháo yào, chuān xiōng, huáng qín,* and *gān cǎo,*
And of *gān lǐ gēn bái pí,* you must consider using a full 200ml!

Commentary 按：

（一）傷寒論云：厥陰之為病，氣上衝心。（二）今奔豚而見往來寒熱，腹痛，是肝臟有邪，而氣通於少陽也。

(1) As the *Shāng Hán Lùn* states, "disease in juéyīn manifests in qì surging up into the heart."
(2) In the present line, running piglet manifests with alternating cold and heat and with abdominal pain. This means that there is evil present in the liver and that the qì has run through to shàoyáng.

Quotation by Wèi Niàntíng 魏念庭云：

（一）上下升降，無論邪正之氣，未有不由少陽，少陽為陰陽之道路也。（二）陰陽相搏則腹痛，氣升則熱，氣降則寒，隨奔豚之氣作患也。

(1) In ascending and descending, downbearing and upbearing, regardless of whether it is evil or right qì, there is none that does not come from shàoyáng. Shàoyáng is the pathway of yīn and yáng.
(2) When yīn and yáng struggle with each other, the result is abdominal pain. When qì is borne upward, heat results. When qì is borne downward, cold results. The trouble arises in accordance with the qì of running piglet.

Quotation by Xú Zhōngkě 徐忠可云：

（一）此方合桂枝、小柴胡二湯，去柴胡，去桂枝，去大棗，以太陽、少陽合病治法，解內外相合之客邪。（二）肝氣不調而加辛溫之芎、歸，熱氣上衝而加苦泄之生葛、李根，不治奔豚，正所以深於治也。

> (1) This formula combines the two decoctions *Guì Zhī Tāng* and *Xiǎo Chái Hú Tāng*, but removes *chái hú, guì zhī*, and *dà zǎo*. It uses a treatment method for combined tàiyáng and shàoyáng disease to resolve the combined internal and external visiting evil. (2) Because liver qì is not harmonized, we add acrid and warm *chuān xiōng* and *dāng guī*; because hot qì is surging upward, we add bitter and discharging *shēng gé* and *gān lǐ gēn bái pí*. [The formula] does not treat running piglet because it directly treats the deeper causes.

Quotation by Yóu Zàijīng 尤在涇云：

芩、桂為奔豚主藥，而不用者，病不由腎發也。

Huáng qín and *guì zhī* are the key medicinals for the treatment of running piglet, and the reason why [the formula] does not use them is that this condition has not arisen from the kidney.[86]

Commentary 按：

服此湯而未愈者，用烏梅丸神效。

If you take this decoction but there is no recovery, using *Wū Méi Wán* has divine efficacy.[87]

86. This formula specifically treats running piglet conditions that originate not in the kidney but in the liver! While it does use *huáng qín*, it does not play the role of sovereign in the present formula.

87. This note was added by a historical commentator of unknown identity.

桂枝加桂湯

Guì Zhī Jiā Guì Tāng

Cinnamon Twig Decoction With Extra Cinnamon

歌見長沙方歌括 。

For the song, see the *Cháng Shā Fāng Gē Kuò*.

治發汗後燒針令其汗，針處被寒，核起而赤者，必發奔豚，氣從少腹上至心，灸其核上各一壯，與此湯主之 。

A treatment for conditions where hot needle therapy after sweating has caused the patient to sweat and the location of the needling therapy has contracted cold, as a result of which a small lump has formed with redness. This situation invariably means that running piglet will erupt, where the qì ascends from the lesser abdomen into the heart. Treat this condition with moxibustion by burning one moxa cone on top of each lump and give this decoction to rule it.[88]

桂枝（ 五兩 ）芍藥（ 三兩 ）甘草（ 二兩，炙 ）生薑（ 三兩 ）大棗（ 十二枚 ）

guì zhī	桂枝		15g
sháo yào	芍藥		9g
gān cǎo	甘草	honey-fried	6g
shēng jiāng	生薑		9g
dà zǎo	大棗		12 pcs

上五味，以水七升，微火煮取三升，去滓，溫服一升 。

Simmer the five ingredients above in 1,400ml of water over gentle heat until reduced to 600ml. Remove the dregs and take 200ml per dose heated.

88. The original formula for *Guì Zhī Tāng* is found in the chapter on Women's Diseases in Pregnancy in the *Jīn Guì Yào Lüè*. The present formula is identical, except for the fact that the amount of *guì zhī* is increased by an additional six grams.

Commentary by [Chén] Yuánxī 元犀按:

（一）汗後又迫其汗，重傷心氣，心氣傷不能下貫元陽，則腎氣寒而水滯也。（二）加以針處被寒，為兩寒相搏，必挾腎邪而凌心，故氣從少腹上至心，發為奔豚也。（三）灸之者，杜其再入之患；用桂枝湯補心氣以解外邪；加桂者，通腎氣，暖水臟，而水邪化矣。

(1) After sweating, if the patient is forced to sweat even more, you double the damage to heart qì, and when heart qì is damaged, it is unable to link up below with original yáng. As a result, kidney qì contracts cold, and water stagnates.
(2) If this situation is then complicated by contraction of cold at the place of needling therapy, the two types of cold struggle with each other and will invariably combine with evil in the kidney to encroach on the heart. For this reason, qì rises up from the lesser abdomen into the heart, and running piglet erupts.
(3) Treating such a patient with moxibustion puts a stop to the problem of repeated invasions. The application of *Guì Zhī Tāng* supplements heart qì to thereby resolve external evil. The additional *guì zhī* frees the flow of kidney qì and warms the water viscus, as a result of which water evil is transformed!

茯苓桂枝甘草大棗湯

Fú Líng Guì Zhī Gān Cǎo Dà Zào Tāng

Poria, Cinnamon Twig, Licorice, and Jujube Decoction

歌見長沙方歌括。

For the song, see the *Cháng Shā Fāng Gē Kuò.*

治發汗後，臍下悸者，欲作奔豚，此湯主之。

A treatment for palpitations below the navel after [the patient has been treated by] promoting sweating, [which indicate that] running piglet is about to break out. This decoction rules it.

茯苓（半斤）甘草（二兩，炙）大棗（十五枚）桂枝（四兩）

fú líng	茯苓		24g
gān cǎo	甘草	honey-fried	6g
dà zǎo	大棗		15 pcs
guì zhī	桂枝		12g

上四味，以甘瀾水一斗，先煮茯苓、減二升，內諸藥，煮取三升，去滓，溫服一升，日三服。

Of the four ingredients above, first simmer the *fú líng* in 2,000ml of potentized water,[89] until reduced by 400ml. Add all the other medicinals and simmer until reduced to 600ml. Remove the dregs and take 200ml per dose heated, three doses per day.

此發汗後心氣不足，而後腎氣乘之，臍下悸，即奔豚之兆也。

This [formula is for patients who,] after sweating, suffer from insufficiency of heart qì, which is then

89. Potentized water, our translation for *gān lán shuǐ* 甘瀾水, is a technical term referring to water that has been lifted and poured with a ladle more than a thousand times. According to Zhāng Zhòngjǐng, this type of water is suitable for treating water evil because the process has altered the medicinal properties of the water. For more information, please refer to Craig Mitchell, Nigel Wiseman, and Feng Ye, *Shāng Hán Lùn* (Paradigm Publications, 1999), p. 170.

exploited by kidney qì and manifests in palpitations below the navel. This is a portent for running piglet.

Commentary from the Sūn Nán Xīn Diǎn Bǐng[90] 孫男心典稟按:

（一）因驚而得，似只宜以心為治也。（二）然自下而上，動於腎氣，激亂於厥陰，而撤守在心，實三經同病也。（三）仲景三方，亦微示其意，學者當隅反之。（四）余讀金匱茯苓桂枝甘草大棗湯治汗後腎氣凌心，即悟桂技甘草湯叉手冒心之治也，更悟桂枝去芍藥加蜀漆牡蠣龍骨救逆湯火逆惊狂之治也。（五）因奔豚湯治氣上衝胸，即悟烏梅丸氣上衝心之治，并四逆散加茯苓，心下悸之治也。（六）因桂枝加桂湯治氣從小腹上衝心，即悟理中湯去朮加佳，臍下動氣之治也。（七）先祖云:仲景書一言一字，俱是活法，難與不讀書者道，亦難與讀書死於句下者道也。

(1) When a condition is contracted because of fright, it appears that we should only treat it in the heart.
(2) Nevertheless, if it ascends from the lower body and stirs kidney qì, irritates juéyīn, and withdraws into the heart, in reality it is the same disease affecting three channels.
(3) In the three formulas above, Zhāng Zhòngjǐng has indicated the meaning only minimally and scholars therefore must deduce it from inference.
(4) Reading in the *Jīn Guì Yào Lüè* that ***Fú Líng Guì Zhī Gān Cǎo Dà Zào Tāng*** treats kidney qì encroaching on the heart after sweating, I immediately realized that ***Guì Zhī Gān Cǎo Tāng*** is a treatment for veiling of the heart [that manifests with the patient] interlocking hands in front of the chest [and applying pressure as the only way to alleviate the discomfort in the heart]. I further realized that ***Guì Zhī Qù Sháo Yào Jiā Shǔ Qī Mǔ Lì Long Gǔ Jiù Nì Tāng*** [rescuing counterflow decoction] is a treatment for fire counterflow with fright and mania.
(5) Because ***Bēn Tún Tāng*** treats qì surging upward into the chest, I realized that ***Wū Méi Wán*** is a treatment for qì surging upward into the heart, and that ***Sì Nì Sǎn*** with the addition of ***fú líng*** is a treatment for palpitations below the heart.
(6) Because ***Guì Zhī Jiā Guì Tāng*** is a treatment for qì surging upward from the lesser abdomen into the heart, I realized that ***Lǐ Zhōng Tāng*** without ***bái zhú*** but with the addition of ***guì zhī*** is a treatment for stirring qì below the navel.
(7) A quotation from an ancestor[91]: Every single sentence and character in Zhāng Zhòngjǐng's writings is describing methods of life. They would be difficult to know for those who didn't study his writings. And they would also be difficult to know for those who did study his writings but died after a sentence.

90. Author and date of this text are unknown.
91. The identity of this "ancestor" is unclear.

胸痹心痛短氣方
Xiōng Bì Xīn Tòng Duǎn Qì Fāng

Formulas for Impediment in the Chest, Heart Pain, and Shortness of Breath

栝蔞薤白白酒湯
Guā Lóu Xiè Bái Bái Jiǔ Tāng
Trichosanthes, Chinese Chive, and White Liquor Decoction

治胸痹病，喘息咳唾，胸背痛，短氣，寸口脈沉而遲，關上小緊數者，此湯主之。

A treatment for conditions of impediment in the chest that manifest with panting and coughing up spittle, pain in the chest and back, shortness of breath, a pulse that is sunken and slow at *cùn kǒu* and small, tight, and rapid above *guān*.[92] This decoction rules it.

栝蔞實（一枚，搗）薤白（半升）白酒（七升）

guā lóu shí	栝蔞實	crushed	1 pc
xiè bái	薤白		100ml
bái jiǔ	白酒		1,400ml

92. As explained in *Nàn Jīng*, Difficult Issue 2, at least one classical school of pulse diagnosis during the *Hàn* period considered two sections for taking the pulse at the wrist, namely the *cùn* ("inch") section (a distance of nine *fēn* from the wrist line to the *guān* "gate") and the *chǐ* ("cubit") section (a distance of one *fēn* from the *guān* upward towards the elbow. For more information, see Unschuld, *Nan-ching* (University of California Press, 1986), pp.81-90. In other contexts, *cùn kǒu* ("inch opening") can also refer to the wrist position in general, which is divided into the three locations *cùn*, *guān*, and *chǐ*, in ascending order from the wrist toward the elbow.

上三味同煮，取二升，分溫再服 。

Simmer the three ingredients above together until reduced to 400ml Divide and take heated in two doses.

Song 歌曰：

胸為陽位似天空，
陰氣彌淪痹不通：
薤白半升栝蔞一個，
七升白酒奏奇功 。

The chest is the position of yáng and resembles the sky.
When yīn qì fully engulfs it, there is impediment and lack of flow.
100ml of *xiè bái* and one piece of *guā lóu shí,*
With 1,400ml of *bái jiŭ* produce a rare effect.

Commentary from the Sūn Nán Xīn Diăn Bĭng 孫男心典稟按：

（一）胸為氣息之路，若陰邪占居其間，則阻其陽氣不通，故生喘息、咳唾、胸背痛諸證。（二）寸口者，脈之大會，陽之位也。（三）內經診脈篇云：上竟上者，胸喉中事也。上附上，右外以候肺，內以候胸中，左外以候心，內以候膻中。（四）此云：寸口脈沉而遲，關上小緊數。寸口，即內經所謂上竟上也。沉為在里，遲為虛寒。（五）關上者，即內經所謂上附上也。緊為陰邪，數為陽氣，顯系胸中陽氣被陰寒痹塞，阻其前後之氣，不相貫通，故見以上种种諸證。（六）方中用栝蔞開胸結，薤白宜心陽，尤妙在白酒散痹通陽，引氣血環環轉身，使前後之氣貫通無礙，則胸中曠若太空，有何胸痹之患戰?

(1) The chest is the pathway for the breath, and if yīn evil occupies its space, it obstructs the yáng qì, preventing it from flowing freely. Therefore the various signs like panting, coughing up spittle, and pain in the back and chest are generated.
(2) *Cùn kŏu* is the great gathering place of the vessels, it is the position of yáng.

(3) As the *Huáng Dì Nèi Jīng* chapter on "Diagnosing Pulses"[93] said, "Above the upper margin[94] [indicates] the affairs in the chest and throat." [It also states,] "Above the uppermost attachment, on the right hand the outside shows the state of the lung and the inside the state inside the chest. On the left hand the outside shows the state of the heart and the inside the state of the pericardiac network vessels."
(4) The present text mentions "a pulse that is sunken and slow at ***cùn kǒu*** and small, tight, and rapid above ***guān***." ***Cùn kǒu*** is precisely what the *Huáng Dì Nèi Jīng* refers to as "above the upper margin." A sunken pulse means that the condition is in the interior, a slow pulse indicates vacuity cold.
(5) Above the ***guān*** is exactly what the *Huáng Dì Nèi Jīng* refers to as "above the upper attachment". Tightness indicates the presence of a yīn evil, and a rapid pulse indicates yáng qì. This illustrates that this condition is related to yáng qì in the chest being impeded by yīn qì, which is obstructing the qì from the front and from behind so that these are unable to link up and flow freely. Therefore we see all the various above-mentioned signs.
(6) In the formula, we use ***guā lóu*** to open up the chest bind, while ***xiè bái*** is well-suited for heart yáng. It is particularly ingenious when mixed into ***bái jiǔ*** to dissipate the impediment [pattern] and free the flow of yáng, drawing qì and blood to circulate continuously all around the body, causing the qì from the front and from behind to link up and flow freely without hindrance. As a result, the space inside the chest is vast like the sky. How could there be any trouble with impediment in the chest?

93. No chapter exists in the *Huáng Dì Nèi Jīng* that is entitled *Zhěn Mài*. Nevertheless, the present quotation comes from *Sù Wèn* 17, which is entitled *Mài Yào Jīng Wéi Lùn* 脈要精微論 (*On the Essential Subtleties of the Pulse*).

94. Indicates the upper edge of the *cùn kǒu* position in pulse diagnosis.

栝蔞薤白半夏湯

Guā Lóu Xiè Bái Bàn Xià Tāng

Trichosanthes, Chinese Chive, and Pinellia Decoction

治胸痹不得臥，心痛徹背者主之 。

A treatment for impediment in the chest with inability to lie down and heart pain penetrating to the back. [This formula] rules it.

栝蔞實（ 一枚，搗 ）薤白（ 三兩 ）半夏（ 半升 ）白酒（ 一斗 ）

guā lóu shí	栝蔞實	crushed	1 pc
xiè bái	薤白		9g
bàn xià	半夏		100ml
bái jiǔ	白酒		2,000ml

上四味同煮，取三升，溫服一升，日三服 。

Simmer the four ingredients above all together until reduced to 600ml. Take 200ml per dose heated, three doses per day.

Song 歌曰：

胸背牽疼不臥時，
上言胸背痛，茲又加以不得臥，其痛甚矣。
所以然者，有痰飲以為之援也。
半升半夏一蔞施，
薤因性濕惟三兩，
即前湯減薤白，只用三兩，惡其濕也。
增入半夏半升，取其燥也。
斗酒同煎滌飲奇 。

When there is pain penetrating from the chest to the back and inability to lie down,
What is above called "pain in the chest and back" is now expanded by "inability to lie down." This means that the pain is severe! The reason for this is that phlegm-rheum is pulling.
Apply 100ml of *bàn xià* and one piece of *guā lóu*,
And because of its damp nature, only nine grams of *xiè bái*.
The amount of *xiè bái* is reduced from the previous decoction: [This formula] uses only nine grams, because its dampness is detestable. Adding 100ml of *bàn xià* takes away its dryness.
Together with 2,000ml of liquor simmer it all, and its results in washing away rheum are rare!

Commentary by [Chén] Yuánxī 元犀按:

加半夏一味，不止滌飲，且能和胃而通陰陽。

The addition of the single ingredient *bàn xià* not only sweeps away rheum but is furthermore able to harmonize the stomach and free the flow of yīn and yáng.

枳實栝蔞薤白桂枝湯

Zhǐ Shí Guā Lóu Xiè Bái Guì Zhī Tāng

Unripe Bitter Orange, Trichosanthes, Chinese Chive, and Cinnamon Twig Decoction

治胸痹，心中痞氣留結在胸，胸滿，脅下逆搶心者，此湯主之。人參湯亦主之。

Impediment in the chest with glomus qì in the heart, being retained and binding in the chest, fullness in the chest, and counterflow below the rib-sides that is scraping against the heart. This formula rules it. *Rén Shēn Tāng* also rules it.

枳實（四枚）薤白（半升）桂枝（一兩）厚朴（四兩）栝蔞實（一枚，搗）

zhǐ shí	枳實		4 pcs
xiè bái	薤白		100ml
guì zhī	桂枝		3g
hòu pò	厚朴		12g
guā lóu shí	栝蔞實	crushed	1 pc

上五味，以水五升，先煮枳、朴，取二升，去滓，入諸藥再煮數沸，分溫再服。

Of the five ingredients above, first simmer the *zhǐ shí* and *hòu pò* in 1,000ml of water until reduced to 400ml. Remove the dregs, add all the other ingredients, and simmer again, bringing it to a boil numerous times. Divide and take heated in two doses.

Song 歌曰：

痞連胸脅逆攻心，
尤云：心下痞氣，是氣痹而成痞也。
按:脅下逆搶心者，氣不由中上而從脅逆，
是中痹而阻諸氣之往來也。

薤白半升四朴尋，
一個栝蔞一兩桂，
四枚枳實撤浮陰。
尤云：宜急通其痞結之氣。

For glomus linking the chest and rib-side and counterflow attacking the heart,
Yóu Zàijīng: "Glomus qì below the heart is glomus formed as the result of qì impediment."
Commentary: Counterflow below the rib-sides that is scraping against the heart means that qì is not rising up from the center but is moving counterflow from the rib-sides. This is impediment in the center that is obstructing all the coming and going of qì.
Seek out 100ml of *xiè bái* and twelve grams of *hòu pò*,
One piece of *guā lóu shí* and three grams of *guì zhī*,
Four pieces of *zhǐ shí* to scatter floating yīn.
Yóu Zàijīng: 'You should urgently free the flow of bound glomus qì.

Commentary by [Chén] Yuánxī 元犀按:

枳實、厚朴泄其痞滿，行其留結，降其搶逆，得桂枝化太陽之氣，而胸中之滯塞自開，以此三藥與薤白、栝蔞之專療胸痹者而同用之，亦去疾莫如盡之旨也。

Zhǐ shí and *hòu pò* discharge the glomus fullness, move the retained and bound [substances], and downbear the scraping counterflow. When [the patient] receives the effect of *guì zhī* in transforming qì in tàiyáng, the stagnation and congestion inside the chest opens up on its own. When you use these three medicinals together with the special efficacy of *xiè bái* and *guā lóu* in curing impediment in the chest, even if [other medicinals] also get rid of the disease, none are as good in their ultimate aim.

人參湯

Rén Shēn Tāng

Ginseng Decoction

即桂枝人參湯。方見傷寒論 。

This is the same as *Guì Zhī Rén Shēn Tāng*. For the formula, see the *Shāng Hán Lùn*."[95]

太阳病，外证未除，而数下之，逐協熱而利，下利不止，心下痞硬，表里不解者，桂枝人參湯主之 。

In tàiyáng disease, when the exterior signs have not yet been eliminated and [the patient has been treated] numerous times with precipitation, resulting in combined heat and diarrhea, with incessant diarrhea, glomus and hardness below the heart, and resolution neither in the exterior nor interior, *Guì Zhī Rén Shēn Tāng* rules.

桂枝四兩 (別切) 甘草四兩 (炙) 白朮三兩 人參三兩 乾薑三兩

guì zhī	桂枝	cut separately	12g
gān cǎo	甘草	honey-fried	12g
bái zhú	白朮		9g
rén shēn	人參		9g
gān jiāng	乾薑		9g

右五味，以水九升，右煮四味，取五升，內桂，更煮取三升，去滓，溫服一升，日再、夜一服 。

Of the five ingredients above, simmer four in 1,800ml of water until reduced to 1,000ml. Add the *guì zhī*, simmer it again until reduced to 600ml, and remove the dregs. Take 200ml per dose heated, two doses per day and one at night.

95. Commentary by unknown editor. For completeness sake, we have added the following formula from the *Shāng Hán Lùn* section on tàiyáng disease, in the chapter on spleen yáng vacuity cold. It is cited there as *Guì Zhī Rén Shēn Tāng*.

Song 歌曰：

理中加桂人參湯，
尤云：速復其不振之陽。
陽復陰邪自散藏，
休訝補攻分兩道，
道消小人道消道長君子道長細推詳。

Center-rectifying Guì Zhī Rén Shēn Tāng
Yóu Zàijīng: "Speedily recovers the devitalized yáng."
Causes yáng to recover and yīn to dissipate on its own among the viscera.
Do not be surprised at the two separate paths of supplementation and attack.
Carefully ponder the path of dispersal **i.e. the path of the "lesser" people**
and the path of growth **i.e. the path of the gentleman.**

Commentary by [Chén] Yuánxī 元犀按：

（一）此別胸痹證虛實之治。（二）實者，邪氣搏結，蔽塞心胸，故不用補虛之品，而專以開泄之劑，使痹氣開則搶逆平矣。（三）虛者，心陽不足，陰氣上彌，故不以開泄之劑，而以溫補為急，使心氣旺則陰邪自散矣。

(1) This is a treatment that differentiates the patterns of impediment in the chest in terms of vacuity and repletion.
(2) In cases of repletion, evil qì is struggling [with right qì] and binding, clouding and congesting the heart and chest. Therefore we do not use substances that supplement vacuity but instead focus on preparations that open and discharge, causing the impediment qì to open, as a result of which the scraping and counterflow are calmed.
(3) In cases of vacuity, heart yáng is insufficient, as a result of which yīn qì engulfs the upper body. Therefore we do not use opening and discharging preparations but instead make warming and supplementing our priority. This causes heart qì to prosper, as a result of which yīn evil dissipates on its own.

Quotation by Yóu Zàijīng 尤在涇云:

（一）去邪之實，即所以安正；補陽之虛，即所以逐陰。（二）是在審其病之久暫，與氣之虛實而決之。

> (1) By removing the repletion of evil, we set right [qì] at ease. By supplementing the vacuity of yáng, we expel yīn.
> (2) While examining the chronic or temporary nature of the disease, we decide by means of the state of vacuity or repletion.

茯苓杏仁甘草湯

Fú Líng Xìng Rén Gān Cǎo Tāng

Poria, Apricot Kernel, and Licorice Decoction

治胸痹，胸中氣塞，短氣者，此湯主之。橘皮枳實生薑湯亦主之。

A treatment for impediment in the chest with qì congestion in the center of the chest and shortness of breath. This decoction rules it. *Jú Pí Zhǐ Shí Shēng Jiāng Tāng* also rules it.

茯苓（三兩）杏仁（五十個）甘草（一兩）

fú líng	茯苓	9g
xìng rén	杏仁	50 pcs
gān cǎo	甘草	3g

上三味，以水一斗，煮取五升，溫服一升，日三服。不差，更服。

Simmer the three ingredients above in 2,00ml of water until reduced to 1,000ml. Take 200ml per dose heated, three doses per day. If there is no recovery, take more.

Song 歌曰：

痹而短氣孰堪醫？
甘一苓三淡泄之，
更有杏仁五十粒，
水行則氣自順不求奇。

Impediment with shortness of qì, who is able to treat it?
Of *gān cǎo* three grams, of *fú líng* nine grams to discharge with blandness.
In addition fifty pieces of *xìng rén,*
When the water moves, qì **naturally** flows smoothly and does not seek out strange [places].

橘皮枳實生薑湯

Jú Pí Zhǐ Shí Shēng Jiāng Tāng

Tangerine Peel, Unripe Bitter Orange, and Fresh Ginger Decoction

橘皮（ 一斤 ）枳實（ 三兩 ）生薑（ 半斤 ）

jú pí	橘皮	48g
zhǐ shí	枳實	9g
shēng jiāng	生薑	24g

上三味，以水五升，煮取二升，分溫再服 。

Simmer the three ingredients above in 1,000ml of water until reduced to 400ml. Divide and take heated in two doses.

Song 歌曰：

痹而氣塞又何施?
枳實辛香三兩宜，
橘用一斤薑減半，
氣開則結自散勿遲疑 。

Impediment and qì congestion, how do you manage this condition?
Of *zhǐ shí's* acridity and fragrance, nine grams are appropriate,
Of *jú pí* use forty-eight grams and of *shēng jiāng* half that amount.
Qì will open up and the bind will dissipate on its own. Do not delay or doubt!

Commentary of teachings received from Lín Lǐfēng[96] 受業林禮豐按：

（一）胸痹胸中氣塞者，由外邪搏動內飲，充塞於至高之分，閉其氣路，非辛溫不能滌飲散邪，非苦泄不能破塞調氣。（二）故重用橘

96. Identity of this person is unknown.

皮、生薑之大辛大溫者，散胸中之飲邪；枳實之圓轉苦辛者，泄胸中之閉塞，譬之寇邪充斥，非雄師不能迅掃也。（三）至若胸痹短氣，乃水邪射肺阻其出氣，只用甘草奠安脾氣，杏仁開泄肺氣，重用茯苓清治節，使水順趨於下，水行而氣自治，譬之導流歸海而橫逆自平也。（四）二方并列，一用辛開，一用淡滲。（五）學者當臨機而酌宜焉。

(1) Impediment in the chest with qì congestion in the center of the chest is caused by external evil striking and stirring internal rheum. It fills up and congests the highest aspect in the body and blocks the pathways of qì there. Without acridity and warmth, we will not be able to wash away rheum and dissipate evil, and without the discharging action of bitterness we will not be able to break up the congestion and harmonize qì.
(2) Therefore by using double amounts of greatly acrid and greatly warm *jú pí* and *shēng jiāng*, we dissipate the rheum evil in the center of the chest. The revolving bitterness and acridity of *zhǐ shí* discharges the blockage in the middle of the chest. We can compare this to a place that is infested with crowds of bandits. If you do not have a mighty army, you will not be able to quickly sweep it clean.
(3) Now if a person suffers from impediment in the chest and shortness of breath, and water evil shoots up into the lung and obstructs the exiting of qì, we use single amounts of *gān cǎo* to settle spleen qì and of *xìng rén* to open up and discharge lung qì, while we use double the amount of *fú líng* to clear management and regulation and cause water to once again flow in its proper direction downward. We can compare the way in which qì regulates itself when water flows to guiding the flow [in flood control] to return to the sea, as a result of which transverse counterflow calms down on its own.
(4) Looking at the two formulas side by side, one uses acridity to open up, and the other uses blandness to percolate.
(5) Students should ponder the appropriateness of these two formulas depending on the particular situation.

薏苡附子散

Yì Yǐ Fù Zǐ Sǎn

Coix and Aconite Powder

治胸痹緩急者，此散主之。

A treatment for impediment in the chest with [alternating] laxness and hypertonicity. This powder rules it.

薏苡仁（十五兩）大附子（十枚，炮）

yì yǐ rén	薏苡仁		45g
dà fù zǐ	大附子	blast-fried	10 pcs

上二味，杵為散，服方寸匕，日三服。

Process the two ingredients above by pestling them into a powder. Take a one gram per dose, three doses per day.

Song 歌曰：

痹來緩急屬陽微，
經云：陽氣者，精則養神，柔則養筋。
附子十枚切莫違，
更有薏仁十五兩，
筋資陰養得陽歸。

Impediment that arrives with [alternating] laxness and hypertonicity is related to yáng debilitation.
The classic states[97]: Yáng qì is delicate to nurture the spirit and is soft to nurture the sinews.
Ten pieces of *fù zǐ*, chopped, do not deviate from this!
Furthermore the formula contains forty-five grams of *yì yǐ rén*.
By supporting the sinews and nurturing yīn, you achieve the return of yáng.

97. This is a famous quote from *Sù Wèn* 3.

Commentary by [Chén] Yuánxī 元犀按:

（一）薏苡稟陽明金氣，金能制風，肝為風臟而主筋，取治筋之緩急，人之所知也。（二）合附子以大補陽氣，其旨甚奧。（三）經云：陽氣者，精則養神，柔則養筋是也。（四）傷寒論桂枝加附子湯與此相表裡。

(1) *Yì yǐ rén* endows metal qì in yángmíng, and metal is able to restrain wind.[98] The liver is the viscus of wind and governs the sinews. Choosing to treat the [alternating] laxness and hypertonicity in the sinews is something that other people also know about.
(2) But combining this with *fù zǐ*, which greatly supplements yáng qì, the meaning of this is extremely profound.
(3) The classic states that "yáng qì is delicate to nurture the spirit and is soft to nurture the sinews."
(4) The formula for *Guì Zhī Jiā Fù Zǐ Tāng* from the *Shāng Hán Lùn* stands in an exterior-interior relationship with this formula.

98. Metal in yángmíng refers to the large intestine. Because wind is wood, metal restrains wind by being able to chop wood.

桂枝生薑枳實湯

Guì Zhī Shēng Jiāng Zhǐ Shí Tāng

Cinnamon Twig, Fresh Ginger, and Unripe Bitter Orange Decoction

治心中痞，諸逆心懸痛者，此湯主之。

A treatment for glomus in the center of the heart with the various types of counterflow and suspension pain in the heart.[99] This decoction rules it.

桂枝生薑（各三兩）枳實（五兩）

guì zhī	桂枝	9g
shēng jiāng	生薑	9g
zhǐ shí	枳實	15g

上三味，以水六升，煮取三升，分溫三服。

Simmer the three ingredients above in 1,200ml of water until reduced to 600ml. Divide and take heated in three doses.

Song 歌曰:

心懸而痛痞相連，
痰飲上彌客氣填；
三兩桂薑五兩枳，
祛寒散逆並攻堅。

Suspension in the heart resulting in pain that is linked to glomus
Means that phlegm-rheum is engulfing the upper body and guest qì is filling in.
Nine grams of *guì zhī* and *shēng jiāng* and fifteen grams of *zhǐ shí*
Repel cold, dissipate counterflow, and attack hardness.

99. The symptom of suspension pain in the heart is explained in the second line of the commentary below.

Commentary by [Chén] Yuánxī 元犀按:

（一）心下痞者，心陽虛而不布，陰邪潛居心下而作痞也。（二）尤云：諸逆，該痰飲、客氣而言。心懸痛者，如空中懸物搖動而痛也。此注亦超。（三）主以桂枝生薑枳實湯者，桂枝色赤，補心壯陽；生薑味辛，散寒降逆；佐以枳實之味苦氣香，苦主泄，香主散，為泄痞散逆之妙品，領薑、桂之辛溫旋轉上下，使陽氣普照，陰邪迅掃而無余耳。

(1) Glomus below the heart means that heart yáng is vacuous and failing to spread out while yīn evil is hiding out below the heart and causing glomus.
(2) Yóu Zàijīng: "All counterflow is describing phlegm-rheum and guest qì. Suspension pain in the heart describes a pain that feels as if caused by something suspended in an empty space and swinging." This note is also outstanding.
(3) Regarding the rulers [among the ingredients] of *Guì Zhī Shēng Jiāng Zhǐ Shí Tāng*, *guì zhī*, being red in color, supplements the heart and strengthens yáng, while *shēng jiāng*, being acrid in flavor, dissipates cold and downbears counterflow. They are assisted by the bitter flavor and fragrant qì of *zhǐ shí*, which is an ingenious substance for discharging glomus and dissipating counterflow, due to the fact that bitterness rules discharge and fragrance rules dissipation. It leads the acrid warmth of *shēng jiāng* and *guì zhī* to cycle all around the upper and lower body. As a result, yáng qì shines into every corner and yīn qì is quickly swept away without any residue being left behind.

烏頭赤石脂丸

Wū Tóu Chì Shí Zhī Wán

Aconite Main Tuber and Halloysite Pill

治心痛徹背，背痛徹心者，此丸主之。

A treatment for heart pain penetrating to the back and back pain penetrating to the heart. These pills rule it.

烏頭（一分，炮）蜀椒乾薑（各一兩）附子（半兩）赤石脂（一兩）

wū tóu	烏頭	**honey-fried**	0.75g
shǔ jiāo	蜀椒		3g
gān jiāng	乾薑		3g
fù zǐ	附子		1.5g
chì shí zhī	赤石脂		3g

上五味末之，蜜丸如桐子大，先食服一丸，日三服。不知，稍加服。

Process the five ingredients above into a powder and form into honey pills the size of firmiana seeds. Take one pill per dose before meals, three doses per day. If you fail to notice any change, slightly increase the dosage.

Song 歌曰：

徹背徹胸痛不休，
前言心痛徹背，尚有止息之時，今則陰寒極而痛極矣。
陽光欲熄實堪憂，
非薤白之類所能治也。
烏頭一分五錢附，
赤石椒薑一兩求。

[In conditions with] incessant pain penetrating to the back and penetrating to the chest
In the above description of "heart pain penetrating to the back" there are times when the

pain desists. In conditions addressed in the present line, the yīn cold is extreme and the pain is extreme as well!

The light of yáng is about to be extinguished, which is truly worthy of great worry
and not a situation that substances like *xiè bái* would be able to cure!
Three-quarters-of-a gram of *wū tóu* and one-and-a-half grams of *fù zǐ*,
Three grams of *chì shí zhī, shǔ jiāo,* and *gān jiāng* must be found!

Quotation by Yù Jiāyán 喻嘉言云:

（一）前後牽連痛楚，氣血疆界俱亂，若用氣分諸藥，轉益其痛，勢必危殆。（二）仲景用蜀椒、烏頭一派辛辣，以溫散其陰邪。（三）然恐胸背既亂之氣難安，而即於溫藥隊中，取用乾薑之守，赤石脂之澀，以填塞厥氣所橫衝之新隊，俾胸之氣自行於胸，背之氣自行於背。（四）各不相犯，其患乃除，此煉石補天之精義也。（五）今人但知有溫氣、補氣、行氣、散氣諸法，不知有填塞邪氣攻衝之竇，令胸背陰陽二氣并行不悖也哉。

(1) Anguishing pain linking the front and the back means that qì and blood in all the border regions are disordered. If you use the various medicinals [that affect] the qì aspect, you will conversely increase the pain, which will invariably create great risk.
(2) Zhāng Zhòngjǐng used *shǔ jiāo* and *wū tóu,* which are both from the group of acrid and spicy medicinals, to warm and dissipate the yīn evil.
(3) Nevertheless, fearing that the disordered qì in the chest and back is difficult to calm, he chose the guarding [effect] of *gān jiāng* and the astringent [effect] of *chì shí zhī* among the squadron of warm medicinals to completely plug up the new tunnel[100] created by the transverse surging of reversal qì, so that the qì from the chest naturally flows in the chest and the qì from the back naturally flows in the back.
(4) Each of these not working against the other and thereby eliminating the trouble, this is the essential meaning of "smelting stones to mend heaven."[101]
(5) People nowadays are only aware that the various methods of warming qì, supplementing qì, moving qì, and dissipating qì exist, but they are not aware of the small opening provided by the technique of "completely plugging up the offensive surging of evil qì." This method causes the two qì of the chest and back and of yīn and yáng to run parallel without conflicting with each other!

100. This quotation, which is also found in other texts like Zhāng Lù's 張璐 *Qiān Jīn Fāng Yǎn Yì* 千金方衍義 (*Expanded Meaning of the Qiān Jīn Fāng*), first published in 1698, appears to suffer from a number of textual corruptions. I read 隊 here as 隧 based on alternate versions of this line.

101. This phrase, coming from an old story about the goddess Nüwa smelting stones in the five colors to patch up heaven, expresses the idea of using supernatural powers to mend a shortcoming.

附方

Fù Fāng

Attached Formulas

九痛丸

Jiǔ Tòng Wán

Nine Pains Pills

（一）治九種心痛：一蟲、二注、三風、四悸、五食、六飲、七冷、八熱、九去來痛是也。（二）而並以一方治之者，豈痛雖有九，其因於各冷結氣者多耶?

(1) A treatment for the nine forms of heart pain, the first being worm [heart pain], the second being influx [heart pain], the third being wind [heart pain], the fourth being palpitations [heart pain], the fifth being food [heart pain], the sixth being drink [heart pain], the seventh being cold [heart pain], the eighth being heat [heart pain], and the ninth being intermittent pain.
(2) Furthermore, regarding the fact that we treat all of these with a single formula, even though there are nine forms, since the cause in each case is cold bound qì, how could there be more [than one treatment]?

附子（三兩，炮）生狼牙 巴豆（去皮，熬，研如膏）乾薑 吳茱萸 人參（各一兩）

fù zǐ	附子	blast-fried	9g
shēng láng yá	生狼牙		3g
bā dòu	巴豆	skin removed, boiled in water, and ground into a paste-like consistency	3g
gān jiāng	乾薑		3g
wú zhū yú	吳茱萸		3g
rén shēn	人參		3g

（一）上六味末之，煉蜜丸如梧桐子大，酒下。（二）強人初服三丸，日三服。（三）弱者二丸。

(1) Process the six ingredients above into a powder and [mix with] refined honey into pills the size of firmiana seeds. Swallow with liquor.
(2) For strong patients, initially take three pills per dose, three doses per day.
(3) For weak patients, take two pills [per dose].

（一）兼治卒中惡，腹脹，口不能言。（二）又治連年積冷，流注心胸痛，並冷衝上氣，落馬，墜車，血疾等證，皆主之。（三）忌口如常法。

(1) These pills are also a treatment for sudden malignity strike with abdominal distention, and inability to speak.
(2) They are also a treatment for cold that has accumulated over a number of years, running and streaming[102] heart and chest pain, as well as for cold surging and qì ascent, falling off a horse or vehicle, blood disease,[103] and similar symptoms. These pills treat them all.
(3) Observe the standard food avoidances.

Song 歌曰:

九種心疼治不難，
狼牙吳萸薑巴豆附參安，
附須三兩余皆一，
攻補同行仔細看。

To treat the nine forms of heart pain is not difficult,
Use *láng yá, wú zhū yú, gān jiāng, bā dòu, fù zǐ,* and *rén shēn* to calm it.
Of *fù zǐ* you need nine grams; of the remaining ingredients three.
Look carefully at applying both the strategies of attack and of supplementation.

102. I.e., flowing around and pooling. The Chinese expression 流注 is also used to refer to the daily movement of qì through the twelve channels, so this phrase could here also mean pain that occurs at different places in accordance with the flow of qì throughout the day.

103. This could quite possibly be a textual error (疾 for 積) and would then mean "blood accumulations."

Quotation by Wèi Niàntíng 魏念庭云:

（一）凡結聚太甚，有形之物參雜其間，暫用此丸。（二）政刑所以濟德禮之窮也。

(1) Whenever bindings and gatherings are too severe and there are tangible things unevenly occurring in various spaces, use these pills intermittently.
(2) Government by punishment is a means of relief in situations where you have reached the limitations of virtue and ritual.

腹滿寒疝宿食方
Fù Mǎn Hán Shàn Sù Shí Fāng

Formulas for Abdominal Fullness, Cold Mounting, and Abiding Food

附子粳米湯
Fù Zǐ Jīng Mǐ Tāng

Aconite and Rice Decoction

治腹中寒氣，雷鳴切痛，胸脅逆滿，嘔吐者，此湯主之。

A treatment for cold qì in the center of the abdomen with thunderous rumbling [in the intestines] and slicing pain, counterflow and fullness in the chest and rib-sides, and retching and vomiting. This decoction rules this condition.

附子（一枚，炮）半夏 粳米（各半升）甘草（一兩）大棗（十枚）

fù zǐ	附子	blast-fried	1 pc
bàn xià	半夏		100ml
jīng mǐ	粳米		100ml
gān cǎo	甘草		3g
dà zǎo	大棗		10 pcs

上五味，以水八升，煮米熟，湯成，去滓，溫服一升，日三服。

Simmer the five ingredients above in 1,600ml of water until the rice is done and the decoction is complete. Take 200ml per dose heated, three doses per day.

Song 歌曰：

腹中切痛作雷鳴，
胸脅皆膨嘔吐成；
附子一枚棗十個，
半升粳夏一甘烹。

For slicing pain in the center of the abdomen and thunderous rumbling,
Both the chest and rib-sides inflated, causing retching and vomiting,
One piece of *fù zǐ* and ten pieces of *dà zǎo,*
100ml of *jīng mǐ* and *bàn xià,* and 3g of *gān cǎo,* cook it all.

Commentary by [Chén] Yuánxī 元犀按：

（一）腹中雷鳴，胸脅逆滿嘔吐，氣也；半夏功能降氣。（二）腹中切痛，寒也；附子功能驅寒。（三）又佐以甘草、粳米、大棗者，取其調和中土，以氣逆為病迸於上，寒生為病起於下，而交乎上下之間者土也。（四）如兵法擊其中堅，而首尾自應也。

(1) Thunderous rumbling in the center of the intestines and counterflow fullness in the chest and rib-sides with retching and vomiting are related to qì. The effect of *bàn xià* is able to downbear qì.
(2) Slicing pain in the center of the abdomen is related to cold. The effect of *fù zǐ* is able to drive out cold.
(3) Moreover, [these ingredients] are assisted by *gān cǎo, jīng mǐ,* and *dà zǎo* because the formula takes advantage of their effect of harmonizing center earth. Given the fact that qì counterflow as a disease bursts forth in the upper body and that the formation of cold as a disease arises in the lower body, the place where they come together in between the upper body and lower body is the center.
(4) This is like the military strategy of striking the hard core, so that the head and tail will follow on their own.

厚朴七物湯

Hòu Pò Qī Wù Tāng

Officinal Magnolia Bark Seven Substances Decoction

治腹滿發熱十日，脈浮而數，飲食如故者，此湯主之。

A treatment for abdominal fullness with with heat erupting for ten days, with a floating and rapid pulse and eating and drinking as usual. This decoction rules this condition.

厚朴（半斤）甘草大黄（各三兩）大棗（十枚）枳實（五枚）桂枝（二兩）生薑（五兩）

hòu pò	厚朴	24g
gān cǎo	甘草	9g
dà huáng	大黄	9g
dà zǎo	大棗	10 pcs
zhǐ shí	枳實	5 pcs
guì zhī	桂枝	6g
shēng jiāng	生薑	15g

（一）上七味，以水一斗，煮取四升，溫服八合，日三服。（二）嘔者加半夏五合；下利去大黄；寒多者加生薑至半斤。

(1) Simmer the seven ingredients above in 2,000ml of water until reduced to 800ml. Take 160ml per dose heated, three doses per day.
(2) For retching, add 100ml of *bàn xià*. For diarrhea, remove the *dà huáng*. For excess cold, increase the amount of *shēng jiāng* to twenty-four grams.

Song 歌曰：

滿而便閉脈兼浮，
三兩甘黄八朴投，

二桂五薑十個棗，
五枚枳實效優優。

For fullness and constipation with the pulse simultaneously being floating,
Toss together nine grams of *gān cǎo* and *dà huáng* and twenty-four grams of *hòu pò*,
Six of *guì zhī*, fifteen of *shēng jiāng*, and ten pieces of *dà zǎo*,
Five pieces of *zhǐ shí*. Truly effective and most outstanding!

Commentary by [Chén] Yuánxī 元犀按:

（一）病過十日，腹滿發熱，脈浮而數。（二）夫脈浮而發熱，邪盛於表也。腹滿而脈數，邪實於里也。（三）表里俱病，故以兩解之法治之。（四）取桂枝湯去芍藥之苦寒，以解表邪而和營衛；小承氣湯蕩胃腸以泄里實。（五）故雖飲食如故，以病已十日之久，表里交病，邪不去則正不复，權宜之法，在所必用也。（六）嘔者，氣逆於上也，故加半夏以降逆；下利去大黃者，以表邪未解，恐重傷胃氣以陷邪也；寒多加生薑者，以太陽本寒之所盛，重用生薑以散寒也。

(1) [In the present case,] the disease has lasted for more than ten days and is manifesting with abdominal fullness, heat effusion, and a floating and rapid pulse.
(2) The floating pulse and heat effusion means that evil exuberates in the exterior. The abdominal fullness and rapid pulse means that evil is replete in the interior.
(3) Since the exterior and interior are both diseased, we treat this condition by the method of dual resolution.
(4) Select *Guì Zhī Tāng* but without the bitter and cold medicinal *sháo yào*, to resolve the evil in the exterior and harmonize construction and defense. And take *Xiǎo Chéng Qì Tāng* to flush the stomach and intestines, thereby discharging the interior repletion.
(5) Because the disease has already persisted for as long as ten days and it is a combined disease of the exterior and interior, even though the patient is drinking and eating as usual, if the evil is not removed, right will not recover. Hence it is necessary to use this stopgap method.
(6) Retching means that qì is moving counterflow in the upper body. Therefore we add *bàn xià* to downbear the counterflow. We remove the *dà huáng* if the patient is suffering from diarrhea because I fear that since the exterior evil is not yet resolved the *dà huáng* will do double damage to stomach qì and thereby trap the evil. We increase the *shēng jiāng* in cases of excessive cold because tàiyáng is the place where the cold is originally exuberant, so we double the amount of *shēng jiāng* to dissipate the cold.

大柴胡湯

Dà Chái Hú Tāng

Major Bupleurum Decoction

歌見長沙方歌括。

For the song, see the *Cháng Shā Fāng Gē Kuò.*

按之心下滿痛者，此為實也，當下之，宜此湯。

Fullness and pain below the heart when you press there means repletion. You must precipitate it, for which this decoction is suitable.

柴胡（半斤）黄芩（三兩）芍藥（三兩）半夏（半升，洗）枳實（四枚，炙）大黄（二兩）大棗（十二枚）生薑（五兩）

chái hú	柴胡		24g
huáng qín	黄芩		9g
sháo yào	芍藥		9g
bàn xià	半夏	washed	100ml
zhǐ shí	枳實	honey-fried	4 pcs
dà huáng	大黄		6g
dà zǎo	大棗		12 pcs
shēng jiāng	生薑		15g

上八味，以水一斗二升，煮取六升，去滓，再煎温服一升，日三服。

Simmer the eight ingredients above in 2,400ml of water until reduced to 1,200ml. Remove the dregs and simmer again. Take 200ml per dose heated, three doses per day.

Commentary by [Chén] Yuánxī 元犀按:

（一）實者當下症，大承氣湯尤恐不及，況大柴胡湯乎？（二）按之心下滿痛者，太陽之邪逆而內干少陽，樞机阻而不利也。（三）用大柴胡湯宜外達內，使少陽之氣從太陽之開而解矣。

(1) In repletion, you must precipitate the concretion. Worrying that *Dà Chéng Qì Tāng* will not reach, what about *Dà Chái Hú Tāng*?
(2) Fullness and pain below the heart when you press there means that the evil in tàiyáng is moving counterflow and internally interfering with shàoyáng.[104] As a result, the mechanism of the pivot is obstructed and inhibited.
(3) Using *Dà Chái Hú Tāng* is suitable for the outside and outthrusts the inside, causing the qì of shàoyáng to be resolved through the opening of tàiyáng.

104. According to *Sù Wèn* 6, shàoyáng is the pivot and tàiyáng is the opening.

厚朴三物湯

Hòu Pò Sān Wù Tāng

Officinal Magnolia Bark Three Substances Decoction

治痛而便閉者，此湯主之 。

A treatment for pain and constipation. This decoction rules it.

厚朴（ 八兩 ）大黄（ 四兩 ）枳實（ 五枚 ）

hòu pò	厚朴	24g
dà huáng	大黄	12g
zhǐ shí	枳實	5 pcs

上三味，以水一斗二升，先煮二味，取五升，內大黄煮取三升，溫服一升，以利為度 。

Of the three ingredients above, first simmer two of them in 2,400ml of water until reduced to 1,000ml. Add the *dà huáng* and simmer again until reduced to 600ml. Take 200ml per dose heated. Use uninhibited movement as your measure [of success].[105]

Song 歌曰：

痛而便閉下無疑，
四兩大黄朴倍之，
枳用五枚先後煮，
小承變法更神奇 。

For pain with constipation below that is beyond doubt,
Twelve grams of *dà huáng* and double that amount of *hòu pò*,

105. When defecation returns to normal and the constipation is cured, you know that the medicine has worked and the patient can stop taking it.

Of *zhǐ shí* five pieces, simmer them in succession.
Being a variation on *Xiǎo Chéng Qì Tāng*, this method is even more marvelous.

Quotation by Yóu Zàijīng 尤在涇云:

（一）承氣意在蕩實，故君大黃。（二）三物意在行氣，故君厚朴。

(1) The intention of *Xiǎo Chéng Qì Tāng* lies in flushing out repletion; hence the sovereign is *dà huáng*.
(2) The intention of *Hòu Pò Sān Wù Tāng* lies in moving qì; hence the sovereign is *hòu pò*.

Commentary by [Chén] Yuánxī 元犀按:

此方不減大黃者，以行氣必先通便，便通則腸胃暢而腑臟氣通，通則不痛也。

The reason this formula does not reduce the amount of *dà huáng* is because to move qì you must first free the stool. When the stool is freed, the intestines and stomach are uninhibited and the qì in the bowels and viscera moves freely. Free flow results in absence of pain.[106]

106. This is a play on words of the famous saying: 不通則痛 (Lack of free flow results in pain).

大承氣湯

Dà Chéng Qì Tāng

Major Qì-Coordinating Decoction[107]

歌見長沙方歌括。

For the song, see the *Cháng Shā Fāng Gē Kuò.*

治腹滿不減，減不足言，當下之。

A treatment for abdominal fullness that does not decrease or decreases only to such an extent that it is not enough to speak of. You should precipitate it.

大黃（四兩，酒洗）厚朴（半升，炙去皮）枳實（五枚，炙）芒硝（三合）

dà huáng	大黃	washed in liquor	12g
hòu pò	厚朴	honey-fried and skin removed	24g
zhǐ shí	枳實	honey-fried	5 pcs
máng xiāo	芒硝		60ml

以上三方，雖緩急不同，而攻泄則一，所謂中滿瀉之於內也。傷寒論淺注已解，毋庸再贅。

Even though the degree of urgency differs between [the conditions treated by] the three formulas above, yet they should all be treated identically by aggressive discharging. This is what is called "[treating] fullness in the center by draining it internally." Since I have already explained this in the *Shāng Hán Lùn Qiǎn Zhù,*[108] there is no need to be redundant.

107. See also above on p.38 and p.248.

108. *Shallow Commentary on the Shāng Hán Lùn* by Chén Xiūyuán published in 1796.

大建中湯

Dà Jiàn Zhōng Tāng

Major Center-Fortifying Decoction

治心胸中大寒痛，嘔不能飲食，腹中滿，上衝皮起，出見有頭足，上下痛而不可觸近者，此湯主之。

A treatment for great cold and pain in the heart and chest, with retching to the point of being unable to drink or eat, fullness in the center of the abdomen that surges upward and makes the skin rise, emerging and looking like head or feet, and pain in the upper and lower body [so severe that] you cannot touch the vicinity of it. This decoction rules it.

蜀椒（二合，炒去汗）乾薑（四兩）人參（二兩）

shǔ jiāo	蜀椒	fried until the sweat is gone	40ml
gān jiāng	乾薑		12g
rén shēn	人參		6g

（一）上三味，以水四升，煮取二升，去滓。（二）內膠飴一升，微火煎取二升，分溫再服。（三）如一炊頃，可飲粥一升，後更服，當一日食糜粥，溫覆之。

(1) Simmer the three ingredients above in 800ml of water until reduced to 400ml. Remove the dregs.
(2) Add 200ml of *jiāo yí* and simmer over a small flame until reduced to 400ml. Divide and take heated in two doses.
(3) After about the time it takes to cook a meal, the patient may drink 200ml of rice gruel and afterwards take another dose. The patient should eat porridge all day long and be covered up warmly.

Song 歌曰:

痛嘔食艱屬大寒，
腹衝頭足觸之難；
腑臟經絡皆寒所痹，痛甚手不可近也。
乾薑四兩椒二合，
參二飴升食粥安 。

Pain with retching and difficulty eating is associated with great cold.
Surging from the abdomen with head and feet that are difficult to touch.
When the bowels and viscera and channels and network vessels are all affected by impediment from cold, the pain is so severe that you cannot get near it with hands.
Twelve grams of *gān jiāng* and 40ml of *shǔ jiāo*,
Six of *rén shēn* and 200ml of *jiāo yí*, along with meals of gruel will quiet [the condition].

Commentary of teachings received from Lín Lǐfēng 受業林禮豐按:

（一）胸為陽氣出入之位。（二）師云：心胸中大寒者，胸中之陽不宣，陰寒之氣從下而上也。（三）痛者，陰寒結聚也。嘔者，陰寒犯胃也。（四）不能食腹中滿者，陰寒犯脾也。（五）上衝皮起，出見有頭足者，陰寒横逆於中也。（六）上下痛而不可触近者是寒從下上，徹上徹下，充滿於胸腹之間，無分界限，陽氣几乎絕滅矣。（七）扼要以圖，其權在於奠安中土。（八）中焦之陽四布，上下可以交泰無虞，故主以大建中湯。（九）方中重用乾薑溫中土之寒；人參、飴糖建中焦之氣；佐以椒性純陽下達，鎮陰邪之逆，助乾薑以振中胃之陽。（十）服後一炊頃飲粥者，亦溫養中焦之氣以行藥力也。

(1) The chest is the location where yáng qì exits and enters.
(2) The teacher said: "If there is great cold in the heart and chest, yáng in the chest is unable to perfuse and the qì of yīn cold ascends from the lower body.
(3) The pain means that yīn cold is binding and gathering. The retching means that yīn cold is invading the stomach.
(4) The inability to eat with fullness in the center of the abdomen means that yīn cold is invading the spleen.
(5) The upward surging that is making the skin rise, emerging and looking like a head or feet, means that yīn cold is moving in transverse counterflow in the center.
(6) Pain in the upper and lower body [so severe that] you cannot touch the vicinity of it means that the cold is ascending from the lower body, penetrating above and penetrating below, and filling up the spaces in the chest and abdomen without knowing any

limits or boundaries, so that yáng qì is nearly expired!
(7) To be concise, [the formula's] power lies in paying respects to and quieting center earth.
(8) When yáng in the middle burner is distributed all over the four directions, above and below are able to join peacefully without worries. Therefore we rule this condition with *Dà Jiàn Zhōng Tāng*.
(9) In the formula, we use double the amount of *gān jiāng* to warm the cold in center earth. *Rén shēn* and *jiāo yí* fortify the qì of the middle burner. They are assisted by *shǔ jiāo*, whose nature is pure yáng and which outthrusts the lower body. Settling the counterflow of the yīn evil, it helps *gān jiāng* in arousing yáng in the stomach at the center.
(10) After taking this medicine, the patient [is instructed to] wait for the amount of time it takes to cook one meal and then drink gruel because this also warms and nourishes the qì of the middle burner and thereby activates the strength of the medicine.

大黃附子湯

Dà Huáng Fù Zǐ Tāng

Rhubarb and Aconite Decoction

治脅下偏痛，脈緊弦，此寒也，以溫藥下之，宜此湯。

A treatment for unilateral pain below the rib-side with a tight string-like pulse. This is a cold [condition]. Use warm medicinals and precipitate it. This decoction is suitable.

大黃（三兩）附子（三枚）細辛（二兩）

dà huáng	大黃	9g
fù zǐ	附子	3 pcs
xì xīn	細辛	6g

（一）上三味，以水五升，煮取二升，分溫三服。（二）若強人，煮取二升半，分溫三服。（三）服後如人行四五裡，進一服。

(1) Simmer the three ingredients above in 1,000ml of water until reduced to 400ml. Divide, and take heated in three doses.
(2) If the patient is a strong person, simmer until reduced to 500ml, divide and take heated in three doses.
(3) After taking it, wait for about the time it takes a person to walk four to five *lǐ*[109] and then take another dose.

109. A *lǐ* is just shy of a mile or slighlty more then half a kilometer.

Song 歌曰：

脅下偏疼脈緊弦，
若非溫下恐遷延；
大黃三兩三枚附，
二兩細辛可補天 。

In cases with unilateral pain below the rib-side and a tight string-like pulse,
If you do not [apply] warmth and precipitation, I fear that the condition will be drawn out.
Nine grams of *dà huáng* and three pieces of *fù zǐ*,
With six grams of *xì xīn* are able to mend heaven.

Quotation by Yóu Zàijīng 尤在涇云:

（一）陰寒成聚，非溫不能已其寒，非下不能去其結。（二）故曰陰寒聚結，宜急以溫藥下之。

(1) When yīn cold forms accumulations, if you do not apply warmth, you will be unable to stop the cold, and if you do not apply precipitation, you will be unable to remove the binds.
(2) Therefore I say: For yīn cold accumulating and binding, you should quickly precipitate by means of warm medicinals.

赤丸方
Chì Wán Fāng
Red Pills Formula

治寒氣厥逆者。

A treatment for cold qì with reverse counterflow.

烏頭（二兩，炮）茯苓（四兩）細辛（一兩）半夏（四兩）

wū tóu	烏頭	blast-fried	6g
fú líng	茯苓		12g
xì xīn	細辛		3g
bàn xià	半夏		12g

（一）上四味末之，內真朱為色，煉蜜為丸，如麻子大。（二）先食飲酒下三丸，日再服。（三）一服不知，稍增，以知為度。

(1) Process the four ingredients above into a powder. Add powdered cinnabar for color and mix with refined honey to form pills the size of hemp seeds.
(2) Before meals, swallow three pills with liquor, two doses per day.
(3) If you do not notice any change after one dose, slightly increase the dosage. Take noticing a change as your measure [of when to stop].

Song 歌曰:

寒而厥逆孰為珍？
四兩夏苓一兩辛，
中有烏頭二兩炮，
蜜丸朱色妙通神。

For cold with reverse counterflow, who holds the gem [of healing]?
Twelve grams of *bàn xià* and *fú líng*, three grams of *xì xīn*,

In their midst six grams of *wū tóu*, blast-fried,
Turned into honey pills the color of cinnabar, what divine ingenuity!

Commentary by [Chén] Yuánxī 元犀按:

（一）寒氣而至厥逆，陰邪盛也。（二）方中烏頭、細辛以溫散獨盛之寒，茯苓、半夏以降泄其逆上之氣，人所共知也。（三）而以朱砂為色，其元妙不可明言，蓋以此品具天地純陽之正色，陽能胜陰，正能勝邪，且以鎮寒氣之浮，而保護心主，心主之令行，則逆者亦感化而效順矣。

(1) Cold qì causing reverse counterflow means that yīn evil is exuberant.
(2) In the formula, *wū tóu* and *xì xīn* dissipate the singly exuberant cold by means of their warming [effect], while *fú líng* and *bàn xià* discharge the counterflow ascending qì by means of their downbearing [effect]. This is common knowledge among the people.
(3) But using cinnabar powder for color, the original subtlety of this strategy is beyond words. Now, this substance is the true color of pure yáng in all of heaven and earth, and yáng is able to defeat yīn and right is able to defeat evil. By settling the floating of cold qì and protecting the heart as the ruler, the commands of the heart as the ruler are carried out. As a result, the counterflow is also transformed in response and the effect is smooth flow.

大烏頭煎

Dà Wū Tóu Jiān

Major Aconite Main Tuber Brew

（一）治腹滿脈弦而緊，弦則衛氣不行，即惡寒；緊則不欲食，邪正相搏，即為寒疝。（二）寒疝繞臍痛，若發則白津出，手足厥冷；其脈沉緊者，此主之。

(1) A treatment for abdominal fullness with a pulse that is stringlike and tight, wherein the stringlike quality means defense qì failing to flow, hence aversion to cold, and the tight quality means lack of appetite and struggle between evil and right, hence the formation of cold mounting.
(2) For cold mounting with pain encircling the navel, and for outbreaks that result in white liquid coming out,[110] reversal cold in the hands and feet, and a sunken and tight pulse, this formula rules.

Commentary by [Chén] Yuánxī 元犀按：

白津者，汗淡不咸，或未睡時泄精漏精，大便下如白痰，若豬脂狀，俱名白津。

White liquid refers to sweat that is bland and not salty, or to discharge or leaking of essence before the patient falls asleep, to defecation of a substance like white phlegm or something that resembles pig lard. All of these are called "white liquid."

烏頭（大者五枚，熬，去皮，不必咀）

wū tóu	烏頭	boiled in water and skin removed, does not need to be pounded	5 large pcs

110. While the text here said "liquid," alternative versions of this formula and [Chén] Yuánxī's note below make it clear that this term here refers to sweat, which is also one of the meanings of *jīn* 津. Moreover, the character 白 here is quite possibly a textual error for 自, which means "spontaneous." See the commentary below.

（一）上以水三升，煮取一升，去滓。（二）内蜜二升，煎令水氣盡，取二升。（三）強人服七合，弱人服五合。（四）不差，明日更服，不可一日更服。

(1) Simmer the ingredient above in 600ml of water until reduced to 200ml and remove the dregs.
(2) Add 400ml of honey and brew until it stops steaming and is reduced to 400ml.
(3) Strong patients should take 140ml per dose, weak patients 100ml per dose.
(4) If the patient fails to recover, take another dose on the next day. You must not take two doses in a single day.

Song 歌曰:

沉緊而弦痛繞臍，
白津汗出淡而不咸之名厥逆四肢冷冷淒淒，一身惡寒之甚。
烏頭五個煮添蜜，
頃刻顛危快挈提。

For a sunken, tight, and string-like pulse with pain encircling the navel,
With [emission of] white liquid **(a name for emission of sweat that is bland and not salty)**,
reverse counterflow **and in the four extremities** severe cold chills
(i.e., severe aversion to cold all over the body),
Simmer five pieces of *wū tóu* and then add honey,
And in a moment the danger will be toppled and the patient rapidly lifted back up [to health].

Commentary by [Chén] Yuánxī 元犀按:

（一）上條與本條，俱陰寒內結之症。（二）寒為厥，氣為逆，是積久陰邪聚滿於中也。（三）陰邪動則氣逆，當為喘嘔不能食矣；陰邪結則阻其陽氣不行，故肢厥膚冷，腹中痛，自汗出矣。（四）曰寒氣厥逆者，乃純陰用事，陽氣將亡，法宜溫中壯陽，大破陰邪。（五）非甘溫辛熱之品，焉能救其萬一哉？

(1) Both the previous paragraph and this one discuss conditions of yīn cold binding internally.
(2) Cold means reversal and qì means counterflow. [Together,] they mean that chronic accumulations of yīn evil are forming gatherings and fullness in the center.

(3) When yīn evil stirs, it results in qì counterflow, which should manifest with panting and retching and inability to eat. When qì evil binds, it obstructs yáng qì and prevents it from flowing, hence we see reversal in the extremities and cold in the skin, pain in the center of the abdomen, and spontaneous sweating.
(4) When the text said "cold qì with reverse counterflow," this means that pure yīn is in charge while yáng qì is about to perish. The appropriate method here is to warm the center and invigorate yáng, and to strongly break up yīn evil.
(5) Without sweet, warm, acrid, and hot substances, how would you be able to rescue even one in a myriad [patients]?

當歸生薑羊肉湯

Dāng Guī Shēng Jiāng Yáng Ròu Tāng

Chinese Angelica, Fresh Ginger, and Goat Meat Decoction

治寒疝腹中痛，及脅痛裡急者，主之。

A treatment for cold mounting with pain in the middle of the abdomen as well as pain in the rib-sides and, and abdominal urgency. [This decoction] rules it.

當歸（三兩）生薑（五兩）羊肉（一斤）

dāng guī	當歸	9g
shēng jiāng	生薑	15g
mutton	羊肉	48g

（一）上三味，以水八升，煮取三升，溫服七合，日三服。（二）若寒多，加生薑成一斤；痛多而嘔者，加橘皮二兩，白朮一兩；加生薑者，亦加水五升，煮取三升二合服之。

(1) Simmer the three ingredients above in 1,600ml of water until reduced to 600ml. Take 140ml per dose heated, three doses per day.
(2) For patients with an excess of cold, increase the amount of *shēng jiāng* to a total of forty-eight grams. For patients with an excess of pain and retching, add six grams of *jú pí* and three grams of *bái zhú*. If you increase the amount of *shēng jiāng*, also increase the amount of water by 1,000ml, simmer until reduced to 640ml, and take that.

Song 歌曰：

腹痛脅疼腹胸皆寒氣作主，無復界限，裡急不堪，是內之營血不足，致陰氣不能相營而急，

羊斤薑五並歸三；

於今豆蔻香砂法，
可笑依盲授指南。

For abdominal pain and pain in the rib-sides **In both the abdomen and chest, cold qì is the ruler, without boundaries or limits,** and abdominal urgency that is unbearable, **This means insufficiency of construction blood on the inside preventing yīn qì from providing construction and causing the urgency.**
Use forty-eight grams of mutton and fifteen of *shēng jiāng* together with nine grams of *dāng guī,*
Concerning the modern method of using *dòu kòu* and *xiāng shā,*
It is laughable to rely on blindness to give guidance.

Song for Modifications 加減歌曰:

寒多增到一斤薑，
痛嘔宜加橘朮商，
朮用一兮橘二兩，
袪痰止嘔補中方。

For excess cold, increase the amount of *shēng jiāng* to forty-eight grams;
For pain with retching, add a share of *jú pí* and *bái zhú,*
Of *bái zhú* use three grams and of *jú pí* six,
A formula to dispel phlegm, stop retching, and supplement the center.

Commentary by [Chén] Yuánxī 元犀按:

（一）方中當歸行血分之滯而定痛，生薑宣氣分之滯而定痛，亦人所共曉也。（二）妙在羊肉之多，羊肉為氣血有情之物，氣味腥羶濃厚，入咽之後即與濁陰混為一家，旋而得當歸之活血而血中之滯通，生薑之利氣而氣中之滯通，通則不痛，而寒氣無有潛藏之地，所謂先誘之而後攻之者也。（三）苟病家以羊肉太補而疑之，是為流俗之說所囿，其中蓋有命焉，知几者即當婉辭而去。

(1) The fact that in this formula *dāng guī* settles pain by moving the stagnation in the blood aspect, and *shēng jiāng* settles pain by diffusing the stagnation in the qì aspect is something that other people also know about.
(2) The ingenuity [of this formula] lies in the large amount of mutton. Mutton is a substance with affinity for qì and blood, its qì and flavor are rank and thick, and after it

enters the back of the throat, it combines with turbid yīn to form one family. Before long, it receives the blood-quickening effect of *dāng guī*, as a result of which the stagnation in the blood aspect is freed. It also receives the qì-disinhibiting effect of *shēng jiāng*, as a result of which the stagnation in the qì aspect is freed. Free flow results in absence of pain, and cold qì does not have a place to lie hidden. This is what is referred to as first luring and then attacking it.

(3) If the patient's family doubts [your actions] on the grounds that mutton is too supplementing, this is because of the limitations of explanations in popular use. Amongst them, you should be the one in command. If you become aware of this at the very beginning, you should diplomatically excuse yourself and leave.

烏頭桂枝湯
Wū Tóu Guì Zhī Tāng
Aconite Main Tuber and Cinnamon Twig Decoction

桂枝湯見傷寒。

For the formula for *Guì Zhī Tāng*, see the *Shāng Hán Lùn.*[111]

（一）治寒疝腹中痛，逆冷，手足不仁。（二）若身疼痛，灸刺諸藥不能治者，抵當烏頭桂枝湯主之。

> (1) A treatment for cold mounting with pain in the center of the abdomen, counterflow cold, and numbness in the hands and feet.
> (2) If there is generalized pain, which moxibustion, acupuncture, and the various medicinals are unable to treat, *Dǐ Dàng Wū Tóu Guì Zhī Tāng* rules it.

烏頭（五枚）（實中者五枚，除去角）蜜（二斤）（千金原年作一斤）
桂枝湯（五合）

wū tóu 烏頭 5 pcs

上一味，以蜜二斤煎減半，去滓，以桂枝湯五合解之，令得一升後，初服五合，不知，即服三合。又不知，复加至五合。其知者如醉狀，得吐者為中病。

Brew the single ingredient above in ninety-six grams of honey until reduced to half and then remove the dregs. Dissolve [the brew] in 100ml of *Guì Zhī Tāng* so that you obtain a total of 200ml. Then initially take 100ml per dose, and if you do not notice any change, take another dose of 60ml. If you still do not notice any change, again increase the dosage up to 100ml. The sign by which you know [that the formula is having an effect] is that the patient appears as if intoxicated. If [the medicine] induces vomiting, this means that it is striking the disease.

111. Craig Mitchell, Nigel Wiseman, and Feng Ye, *Shāng Hán Lùn* (Paradigm Publications, 1999), chapter 1, pp. 61-62.

Song 歌曰：

腹痛內寒身疼外寒肢不仁，脾主四肢，
不仁者，寒盛於中，無陽氣以溫之也。
藥攻刺灸治非真，
或攻其內，或攻其外，邪氣牽制不服，
而可以抵當其病者，惟有本方。
桂枝湯照原方煮，
蜜煮烏頭合用神。

For abdominal pain **(internal cold)**, generalized pain **(external cold)**, and numbness
in the extremities **(the spleen rules the four extremities and when they are numb,
it means that cold is exuberant in the center and that there is no yáng qì to warm it.)**
When neither attack with medicinals nor treatment with acupuncture or moxibustion
produce true results **(whether you attack the inside or the outside,
if evil qì cannot be curbed, it is only with this formula that you can resist the disease.)**
Simmer *Guì Zhī Tāng* according to the original formula,
Mix with *wū tóu* and simmer in honey for divine effects.

Commentary 按：

解之者，溶化也。知，效也。如醉狀，外寒方解。得吐者，內寒已伸，故為中病也。

"Dissolve" means to melt. "The sign by which you know" means the effect. "Appearing as if intoxicated" means that the external cold is just then being resolved. "If the medicine induces vomiting" means that the internal cold is already stretched, hence it means that it is striking the disease.

（一）道光庚辰歲，予大小兒年二十六歲，初病時少腹滿，兩旁相去有六寸遠結二癰，長三寸，闊二寸，不紅不痛，其氣似相通狀，大便不通，發作寒熱，食少。（二）醫者紛紜不一，或以托裡發散，或用下法，藥多不效。（三）至二三日之後，少腹滿，漸高脹及腹上，及胸脅，逆氣衝及咽喉，藥物飲食不能下咽，氣喘，冷汗出，四肢厥，有一時許竟目直口開。（四）予不得已，用大溫回陽之劑灌之，其初不能下咽，後約進有四分之一，其氣略平些，蘇回。（五）予查其病症，云夜夜泄精，或有夢，或無夢，泄時知覺，以手捏之，有二三刻久方止，夜夜如是，後驚不敢睡，至雞鳴時亦泄，診其脈弦細芤遲。

（六）余思良久，方覺陰寒精自出句，生二癰者，乃陰寒聚結也。（七）治之非大溫大毒之品，不能散陰寒之結；非大補元氣，不能勝陰邪之毒也。（八）後用四逆、白通、理中、建中等湯數服，病症漸漸而差。（九）此足見長沙之法，運用無窮。願後之學者，深思而自得焉可。

(1) In the *gēng-chén* year of the reign period Dào-Guáng,[112] my eldest child of twenty-six years, when first falling ill, suffered from fullness in the lesser abdomen with two welling-abscesses on both sides, separated from each other by a distance of about six *cùn*, that were three *cùn* in length and two *cùn* in width. Neither red nor painful, their qì seemed to be connected to each other, [and the condition was accompanied by] stopped defecation, intermittent cold and heat, and reduced eating.
(2) The physicians treated the condition with a confused and varied array of approaches, some by means of internal expulsion, effusing and dissipating, and some by using precipitation. The medicinals were many but all without effect.
(3) Two or three day after that, the fullness in the lesser abdomen gradually rose higher and turned into distention reaching to above the abdomen, then reaching the chest and rib-sides, with counterflow qì surging into the throat, so that neither medicinal substances nor drink or food could go down his throat, with panting, discharge of cold sweat, reversal in the four extremities, and even causing suddenly forward-staring eyes and open mouth at one time.
(4) I had no other alternative but to use a strongly warming and yáng-returning preparation and pour it into him. Initially, it was impossible to get it down the throat, but then I gradually managed to get a quarter of it in. The patient's qì became slightly more calm and he was revived.
(5) I checked with the patient for pathological symptoms and he said that he had been experiencing seminal discharge night after night, sometimes in his dreams and sometimes without dreaming. At the time of discharging, he could feel a sensation and would use his hands to knead it. After two or three quarter hours it would stop. Night after night was like this. Subsequently, he had grown so alarmed that he did not dare to fall asleep, but even waiting up until the time of the rooster crowing, he would still have the discharge. I examined his pulse and found it to be stringlike, fine, scallion-stalk, and slow.
(6) I thought about it for a good length of time and then felt that yīn cold was causing essence to discharge spontaneously. The formation of the two welling-abscesses was in fact a case of yīn cold gathering and binding.
(7) In treatment, without strongly warming and strongly toxic substances, we would be unable to dissipate the binding of yīn cold, and without strongly supplementing original qì, we would be unable to overcome the toxin of yīn evil.
(8) Subsequently I used numerous doses of decoctions like *Sì Nì Tāng*, *Bái Tōng Tāng*,

112. I.e., 1821 C.E.

Lǐ Zhōng Tāng, and *Jiàn Zhōng Tāng*, and the symptoms of the illness were gradually cured.
(9) This [example] is enough to see the method of [Zhāng Zhòngjǐng from] Cháng Shā with its limitless applications. I hope that later students will contemplate this deeply and become capable by grasping it on their own.

附方
Fù Fāng
Attached Formulas

外台烏頭湯
Wài Tái Wū Tóu Tāng
Aconite Main Tuber Decoction from the *Wài Tái Mì Yào*

（一）治寒疝，腹中絞痛，賊風入攻，五臟拘急，不得轉側，發作有時，令人陰縮，手足厥逆。（二）即大烏頭煎。（三）方見上。

(1) A treatment for cold mounting, with gripping pain in the abdomen, bandit wind entering and attacking, hypertonicity in the five viscera, inability to turn to the side, symptoms occurring at set times, causing the person's genitals to contract, and reverse counterflow in the hands and feet.
(2) This is identical with *Dà Wū Tóu Jiān.*
(3) For the formula, see above.[113]

113. See p. 233 above.

外台柴胡桂枝湯

Wài Tái Chái Hú Guì Zhī Tāng

Bupleurum and Cinnamon Twig Decoction from the *Wài Tái Mì Yào*

歌見長沙方歌括。

For the song, see the *Cháng Shā Fāng Gē Kuò.*

治心腹卒中痛者。

A treatment for sudden strike in the heart or abdomen with pain.

柴胡（四兩）黃芩（一兩半）人參（一兩半）半夏（二合半）大棗（十二枚）生薑（三兩）甘草（一兩）桂枝（一兩半）芍藥（一兩半）

chái hú	柴胡	12g
huáng qín	黃芩	4.5g
rén shēn	人參	4.5g
bàn xià	半夏	50ml
dà zǎo	大棗	12 pcs
shēng jiāng	生薑	9g
gān cǎo	甘草	3g
guì zhī	桂枝	4.5g
sháo yào	芍藥	4.5g

上九味，以水六升，煮取三升，溫服一升，日三服。

Simmer the nine ingredients above in 1,200ml of water until reduced to 600ml. Take 200ml per dose heated, three doses per day.

外台走馬湯

Wài Tái Zǒu Mǎ Tāng

Galloping Horse Decoction from the *Wài Tái Mì Yào*

治中惡心痛腹脹，大便不通。

A treatment for malignity strike with heart pain and abdominal distention and stopped defecation.

巴豆（二枚，去皮心，熬）杏仁（二枚）

bā dòu	巴豆	skin and core removed, boiled in water	2 pcs
xìng rén	杏仁		2 pcs

上二味，以綿纏捶令碎，熱湯二合，捻取白汁飲之，當下。老少量之，通治飛尸、鬼擊病。

Wrap the two ingredients above in gauze and pound until crushed. Place in 40ml of hot water and wring out to obtain a white liquid. Drink this. It should cause precipitation. For elderly [patients], reduce the amount. It is also a treatment for the diseases of flying corpse and being beaten by demons.[114]

Song 歌曰：

外來異氣傷人多，
腹脹心疼走馬搓；
巴杏二枚同搗細，
衝湯捻汁好驅邪。

When strange qì coming from the outside damages a person excessively,
[Manifesting in] abdominal distention and heart pain, galloping horse [decoction] will rub it [out].
Two pieces each of *bā dòu* and *xìng rén*, pounded until fine,

114. See footnote above on Corpse syndrome, on p. 152.

Rinsed with hot liquid and wrung out, the liquid is good for driving out evil.

Commentary of teachings received from the disciple of Lín Shìyōng[115] 受業門人林士雍按：

（一）中惡心痛，大便不通，此實邪也。（二）然邪氣雖實，亦以體虛而受也，是故有虛實寒熱之异，不得執一說而定之。（三）仲師附走馬湯者，以巴豆辛溫大毒，除鬼注蠱毒，利水谷道；杏仁甘、苦、溫，有小毒，入肺經，肺為天，主皮毛，中惡腹脹滿者，以惡毒不离皮毛口鼻而入，故亦從皮毛高原之處而攻之，以毒攻毒，一鼓而下也。（四）此附治寒實大毒之邪，氣虛者則不可用矣。（五）近世有痧疾病，疑即此也。（六）昔聞之先業師曰：今所謂痧疾者，乃六淫邪毒猛惡厲氣所傷，凡所過之處，血氣為之凝滯不行，其症或見身痛，心腹脹滿絞痛；或通身青紫，四肢厥冷，指甲色如靛青，口噤，牙關緊閉，不能言語；或心中忙亂，死在旦夕，是邪毒內入矣。（七）宜瀉其毒，或刺尺澤、委中、足十趾，必使絡脈貫通，氣血流行，毒邪自解矣。（八）愚意：輕者用刮痧之法，隨即服紫金錠，或吐或下或汗出，務使經氣流通，毒邪亦解；或吐瀉不止，腹痛肢厥，大汗出，脈微欲絕者，宜用白通湯、通脈四逆湯、四逆湯等，以回陽氣，以化陰邪，庶毒厲之邪漸消。（九）若口不能開者，當從鼻孔中灌之。

(1) Malignity strike with heart pain and stopped defecation, this means a repletion of evil.
(2) Now even though the evil qì is replete, it is at the same time contracted as the result of vacuity in the body. For this reason, there is a difference between vacuity and repletion and cold and hot and you must not hold onto only a single theory to determine the [proper course of action].
(3) The reason Zhāng Zhòngjǐng attached [the formula for] *Zǒu Mǎ Tāng* here is that *bā dòu* is acrid and warm and greatly toxic, eliminates demonic infixation and *gǔ* toxin, and disinhibits the pathways of water and grain. *Xìng rén* is sweet, bitter, warm, and slightly toxic. It enters the lung channel. Since the lung is heaven and rules the skin and body hair, if patients suffer from malignity stroke with abdominal distention and fullness and the malignity evil has entered through the mouth and nose not far from the skin and body hair, you can therefore also attack it from the place that is the highest source of the skin and body hair. Using toxin to attack toxin, you will precipitate it with a single drumbeat.

115. Identity of this person is unknown.

(4) This attached formula is a treatment for cold repletion with evil of great toxicity. In patients with qì vacuity, you may not use it!

(5) In our modern times, we have the condition of sand disease, and I wonder if this is not identical with it.

(6) I heard my late teacher say: What we now refer to as sand disease in fact refers to damages from the six excesses, evil toxins, fierce malignity, and pestilential qì. In all the places where these are in excess, blood and qì congeal and stagnate instead of flowing. In terms of the symptoms, you may see pain in the body with distention, fullness and gripping pain in the heart and abdomen; or possibly blue-green and purple coloration running through the body, reversal cold in the four extremities, a color in the finger nails like indigo blue, clenched mouth, teeth locked tight, and inability to speak; or possibly fussing and confusion in the heart, followed shortly by death. This is the evil toxin entering the inside of the body.

(7) It is appropriate to drain the toxin, possibly by piercing[116] *Chǐ Zé* (LU-5), *Wěi Zhōng* (BL-40), and the ten toes. You must penetrate to the network vessels and restore the flow of qì and blood, and the evil will resolve on its own.

(8) My humble opinion: In mild cases, use the method of *guā shā*,[117] immediately followed by ingesting *Zǐ Jīn Dìng*.[118] Whether you induce vomiting or precipitation or sweating, make sure that the qì in the channels is flowing freely and the toxic evil will also resolve. Alternatively, if the patient is suffering from incessant vomiting and diarrhea, abdominal pain and reversal in the extremities, severe sweating, and a faint pulse about to expire, it is suitable to use *Bái Tōng Tāng*, *Tōng Mài Sì Nì Tāng*, *Sì Nì Tāng*, etc., to make yáng qì return and to transform yīn evil, thereby gradually making the numerous evils of toxic pestilence disappear.

(9) If you are unable to open the patient's mouth, pour it in through the nostrils.

116. In the present context, the character 刺 does not mean to apply fine acupuncture needles in the modern sense of the term, but rather to make the patient bleed at these points, in order to remove the toxins.

117. Literally translated, this term means "sand-scraping."

118. Literally meaning "purple gold bullion," this term is an alternate name for *Yù Shū Dān* 玉樞丹 (Jade Pivot Pills), a preparation made of *shè xiāng* 麝香, *zhū shā* 朱砂, *xióng huáng* 雄黃, *dà jǐ* 大戟, *wǔ bèi zǐ* 五倍子, *shān cí gū* 山慈姑, etc.

A quotation from the *Jí Yàn Liáng Fāng*[119] 集驗良方有云:

（一）行路之人，路中犯此痧疾者，不得不用刮痧之法。（二）刮後或其人不省者，宜用人尿拌土，將此土環繞臍中，復使同行之人向臍中溺之，使中宮溫，則氣機轉運，血脈流行矣。

(1) When a person just walking along a road in the middle of the road is attacked by this sand disease, you must absolutely apply the *guā shā* technique.
(2) After scraping, if the patient is unconscious, it is good to use human urine and mix it with some dirt. Take this dirt and spread it all around the navel. Then make a person who has walked the same path urinate on the center of the [patient's] navel, causing the central palace to become warm. As a result the qì dynamic will turn around and move and the blood in the vessels will flow freely!

119. *Excellent Formulas from Collected Experience.* While not absolutely certain, this title most likely refers to a text that is elsewhere referred to as *Jí Yàn Fāng* 集驗方 (*Formulas from Collected Experience*). Quoted for example in the medieval collection *Yī Xīn Fāng* 醫心方 more than 130 times, it was composed in the sixth century by Yáo Sēngyuán 姚僧垣.

大承氣湯

Dà Chéng Qì Tāng

Major Qì-Coordinating Decoction[120]

歌見傷寒淺注

For the song, see the *Shāng Hán Qiǎn Zhù*.

(一) 寸口脈浮而大，按之反澀，尺中亦微而澀者，有宿食也 。此湯主之 。(二) 數而滑者，實也，此有宿食，下之愈，宜此湯 。(三) 下利不欲食者，此有宿食，當下之，宜此湯 。

(1) A treatment for a pulse that is floating and large at ***cùn kǒu*** but when pressed on the contrary rough. A pulse that is faint and rough in the ***chǐ*** position[121] as well means the presence of abiding food. This decoction rules it.
(2) A rapid and slippery pulse means repletion. This means the presence of abiding food. Precipitating it will cure the condition. This decoction is appropriate.
(3) When there is diarrhea and no desire for food, this means the presence of abiding food. You should precipitate it. This decoction is appropriate.

120. For the formula instructions and discussion, see also p.38 and p.225.

121. See the explanatory footnote to pulse positions on p. 195 above.

栝蒂散

Guā Dì Sǎn

Melon Stalk Powder[122]

歌見長沙方歌括。

For the song, see the *Cháng Shā Fāng Gē Kuò*.

治宿食在上脘，當吐之，宜此散主之。

A treatment for abiding food in the upper stomach duct. You should [treat it] by inducing vomiting. This powder is appropriate to rule it.

122. See also p.54 above for the formula and indications on *Guā Dì Sǎn*.

Pinyin	Character	Botanical name	Common Name
bā dòu	巴豆	Seed of Croton tiglium	croton
bái jiǔ	白酒		white liquor
bái liǎn	白蘞	Root of Ampelopsis japonica	ampelopsis root
bái qián	白前	Root and rhizome of Cynanchum stauntoni	willowleaf swallowwort root and rhizome
bái shí zhī	白石脂	Kaolin	China clay
bái wēi	白薇	Root of Cynanchum atratum	black swallowwort root
bái zhú	白朮	Rhizome of Atractylodes macrocephala	white atractylodes rhizome
bǎi hé	百合	Bulb of Lilium brownii	trumpet lily bulb
bàn xià	半夏	Rhizome of Pinellia ternata	pinellia rhizome
bèi mǔ	貝母	Bulb of Fritillariae cirrhosa	fritillaria bulb
biē jiǎ	鱉甲	Dorsal shell of Amyda sinensis	turtle shell
chái hú	柴胡	Root of Bupleurum chinense	bupleurum root
cháng shān	常山	Root of Dichroa febrifuga	dichroa root
chì shí zhī	赤石脂	Halloysite	halloysite
chì xiāo	赤硝	Niter	niter
chì xiǎo dòu	赤小豆	Fruit of Phaseolus calcaratus	aduki/rice bean
chuān xiōng	川芎	Root of Ligusticum wallichii	chuanxiong root
dà fù zǐ	大附子	Lateral root of Aconitum carmichaeli	aconite lateral root
dà huáng	大黃	Root of Rheum palmatum	rhubarb root
dà jǐ	大戟	Root of Euphorbia pekinensis	Peking spurge root
dà zǎo	大棗	Mature fruit of Ziziphus jujuba	jujube
dài zhě shí	代赭石	Hematite	hematite
dāng guī	當歸	Root of Angelica sinensis	Chinese angelica root
dòu huáng juǎn	豆黃卷	Dried sprout of Glycines max	dried soy bean sprout
dú huó	獨活	Root and rhizome of Angelica pubescens	pubescent angelica root
ē jiāo	阿膠	Gelatinous glue produced from Equus asinus	donkey-hide gelatin
fán shí	礬石	Alum	alum
fáng fēng	防風	Root of Ledebouriella divaricata	saposhnikovia root
fáng jǐ	防己	Root of Aristolochia fangchi or Stephania tetranda	fangji root

fēng fáng	蜂房	Nest of Vespa	hornet's nest
fēng wō	蜂窠	Nest of Vespa	hornet's nest
fú líng	茯苓	Dried fungus of Poria cocos	poria
fù zǐ	附子	Lateral root of Aconitum carmichaeli	aconite lateral root
gān cǎo	甘草	Root of Glycyrrhiza uralensis	licorice root
gān dì huáng	乾地黄	Dried root of Rehmannia glutinosa	dried rehmannia root
gān jiāng	乾薑	Dried root of Zingiber officinale	dried ginger
gān lǐ gēn bái pí	甘李根白皮	Root of Prunus salicina	Chinese plum root bark
gān qī	乾漆	Dried sap of Rhus verniciflua	lacquer
gé gēn	葛根	Root of Pueraria lobata	kudzu root
guā bàn	瓜瓣	Seed of Benincasa hispida	wax gourd/winter melon seed
guā dì	瓜蒂	Stalk of Cucumis melo	muskmelon stalk
guā lóu gēn	栝蔞根	Root of Trichosanthes kirilowii	trichosanthes root
guā lóu shí	栝蔞實	Fruit of Trichosanthes kirilowii	trichosanthes fruit
guì zhī	桂枝	Twigs of Cinnamomum cassia	cinnamon twig
hǎi zǎo	海藻	Sargassum fusiforme	sargassum
hán shuǐ shí	寒水石	Sodium calcium sulfate	glauberite
hòu pò	厚朴	Bark of Magnolia officinalis	officinal magnolia bark
huá shí	滑石	Talcum	talcum
huái bái pí	槐白皮	Root bark of Sophora japonica	Pagoda tree root bark
huáng lián	黄連	Rhizome of Coptis chinensis	coptis rhizome
huáng qí	黄芪	Root of Astragalus membranaceus	astragalus root
huáng qín	黄芩	Root of Scutellaria baicalensis	Chinese skullcap root
jī zǐ huáng	雞子黄	Egg yolk of Gallus gallus domesticus	egg yolk
jiāo yí	膠飴	Malt candy	malt candy
jié gěng	桔梗	Root of Platycodon grandiflorum	balloon flower root
jú pí	橘皮	Peel of Citrus reticulata	tangerine peel
kǔ shēn	苦參	Root of Sophora flavescens	flavescent sophora root
kuǎn dōng huā	款冬花	Flower of Tussilago farfara	coltsfoot flower
láng yá gēn	狼牙根	Root of Potentilla cryptotaenia/Agrimonia pilosa	cinquefoil/downy agrimony root
lóng gǔ	龍骨	Mastodi Ossis Fossilia	dragon bone (i.e. fossilized mastodon bones)
lú rú	藘茹	Rubia cordifolia	madder root
má huáng	麻黄	Stalk of Ephedra sinica	ephedra stalk

mài mén dōng	麥門冬	Tuber of Ophiopogon japonicus	ophiopogon/Japanese hyacinth tuber
máng xiāo	芒硝	Hydrated sodium sulfate	pure mirabilite
méng chóng	虻蟲	Tabanus	female gadfly
mì	蜜	Honey of Apis cerana	honey
mǔ dān pí	牡丹皮	Bark of the root of Paeonia suffruticosa	tree peony root bark
mǔ lì	牡蠣	Shell of Ostrea rivularis	oyster shell
qí cáo	蠐螬	Dried larva of Holotrichia diomphalia	Korean black chafer grub
qiāng láng	蜣螂	Catharsius	dung beetle
qū mài	瞿麥	Entire plant, including flowers, of Dianthus superbus	dianthus plant
rén shēn	人參	Root of Panax ginseng	ginseng root
shān zhū yú	山茱萸	Fruit of Cornus officinalis	cornus/dogwood fruit
sháo yào	芍藥	Root of Paeonia albiflora	peony root
shè gān	射乾	Rhizome of Belamcanda chinensis	belamcanda/leopard lily rhizome
shén qū	神曲/麴	Medicated leaven	medicated leaven
shēng dì huáng zhī	生地黃汁	Juice from the fresh root of Rehmannia glutinosa	fresh rehmannia root juice
shēng gé	生葛	Fresh Puerariae	
shēng jiāng	生薑	Fresh root of Zingiber officinale	fresh ginger
shēng láng yá	生狼牙	Fresh leaf of Agrimoniae	
shēng má	升麻	Rhizome of Cimifuga foetida	cimicifuga/cohosh rhizome
shí gāo	石膏	Gypsum	gypsum
shí wéi	石韋	Foliage of Pyrrosia lingua	pyrrosia leaf
shǔ fù	鼠婦	Dried body of Armadillidium vulgare	pill bug/woodlouse/roly-poly
shǔ jiāo	蜀椒	Seed capsules of Zanthoxylum bungeanum	zanthoxylum seed capsule
shǔ qī	蜀漆	Foliage of Dichroa febrifuga	dichroa leaf
shǔ yù	薯蕷	Root of Dioscorea opposita	diosorea rhizome/potato yam
shuǐ zhì	水蛭	Dried body of Whitmania pigra	leech
suān zǎo rén	酸棗仁	Seed of Ziziphus spinosa	spiny jujube seed
táo rén	桃仁	Seed of Prunus persica	peach pit
tián guā dì	甜瓜蒂	Stalk of Melonis	sweet guā dì
tiān huā fěn	天花粉	Root of Trichosanthis kirilowii	trichosanthes root
tiān xióng	天雄	Mature root of Aconitum carmichaeli	tianxiong aconite root
tíng lì	葶藶	Seed of Lepidium apetalum or Descurainia	pepperwort or descurainia seed.

wěi jīng	葦莖	Stem of Phragmititis caulis	phragmites stem
wū shàn	烏扇	Rhizome of Belamcanda chinensis	belamcanda/leopard lily rhizome
wū tóu	烏頭	Main tuber of Aconitum carmichaeli	aconite main tuber
wū zéi gǔ	烏鰂骨	Bone of Sepialla maindroni	cuttlefish bone
wú zhū yú	吳茱萸	Unripe fruit of Evodia rutaecarpa	evodia
wǔ wèi zǐ	五味子	Fruit of Schisandra chinensis	schisandra fruit
xì xīn	細辛	Complete plant including root of Asarum heteropoides	asarum/wild ginger
xiāng chǐ	香豉	Preparation of Fermented Glycine max	fermented soybean
xiǎo mài	小麥	Seed of Triticum aestivum	wheat
xiè bái	薤白	Stalk of Allium macrostemon	Chinese chive
xìng rén	杏仁	Dried seed of Prunus armeniaca	apricot pit
xióng huáng	雄黃	Realgar	realgar
yán	鹽	Sodium chloride	salt
yáng ròu	羊肉	Meat of Capra hircus or Ovis aries	mutton
yí táng	飴糖		malt sugar
yì yǐ rén	薏苡仁	Seed kernel of Coix lachryma-jobi	Job's tears
yún mǔ	雲母	Muscovite	muscovite
zào jiá	皂莢	Fruit of Gleditsia sinensis	gleditsia/honey locust fruit
zé qī	澤漆	Entire plant of Euphorbia helioscopia	sun spurge
zé xiè	澤瀉	Rhizome of Alisma plantago-aquatica	alisma rhizome
zhè chóng	蟅蟲	Entire dried body of the female of Eupolyphaga sinensis	ground beetle
zhī mǔ	知母	Root of Anemarrhena asphodeloides	anemarrhena root
zhǐ shí	枳實	Unripe fruit of Poncirus trifoliata or Citrus aurantium	unripe Chinese hardy orange or bitter orange
zǐ shēn	紫參	Salvia chinensis	Chinese salvia plant
zǐ shí yīng	紫石英	Fluorite	fluorite
zǐ wǎn	紫菀	Root and rhizome of Aster tataricus	aster root
zǐ wēi	紫葳	Flower of Campsis grandiflora	campsis/Chinese trumpet flower

Formulas, Indications, and Actions

Excerpted from the 1921 edition of the *Zhōng Guó Yī Xué Dà Cí Diǎn* 中國醫學大辭典 (*Great Dictionary of Medicine in China*) and arranged in the order in which the formulas occur in the source text.

栝蔞桂枝湯
Guā Lóu Guì Zhī Tāng

guā lóu gēn	栝蔞根	9g
guì zhī	桂枝	9g
shēng jiāng	生薑	9g
sháo yào	芍藥	9g
gān cǎo	甘草	6g
dà zǎo	大棗	12 pcs

Indications: Tetany disease in the tàiyáng channel.

Analysis:

- *Guì Zhī Tāng* with the addition of *guā lóu gēn*.
- Complete range of tàiyáng symptoms makes it evident that the evil is in the exterior.
- Slow and sunken pulse indicates that this evil is caused by internal exhaustion of fluids.
- Treat not by exterior dissipation of wind-cold but by clearing heat in the qì aspect and engendering liquids (*guā lóu gēn*), and harmonizing construction and defense (*guì zhī*).

葛根湯
Gé Gēn Tāng

gé gēn	葛根	12g
má huáng	麻黄	9g
guì zhī	桂枝	6g
sháo yào	芍藥	6g
shēng jiāng	生薑	9g
dà zǎo	大棗	12 pcs
gān cǎo	甘草	6g

Indications: Combined tàiyáng and yángmíng disease, possibly with diarrhea or retching, turning into reduced urination; heat effusion but no sweating; panting, fullness, and no eating; clenched mouth and inability to speak; about to erupt as hard tetany.

Analysis:

- *Guì Zhī Tāng* with the addition of *má huáng* and *gé gēn*.
- Treats tàiyáng disease that is unresolved and has moved into yángmíng.
- *Gé gēn* is the sovereign because it courses yángmíng and clears the fleshy exterior, thereby eliminating both the internal signs of retching and diarrhea and the external signs of clenched mouth and heat in the skin.
- *Má huáng* courses lung qì and frees the flow in the skin and body hair, resolving internal panting and fullness and external absence of sweating.

大承氣湯
Dà Chéng Qì Tāng

dà huáng	大黃	12g
hòu pò	厚朴	24g
zhǐ shí	枳實	5 pcs
máng xiāo	芒硝	60 ml

Indications: Yángmíng repletion heat patterns, with dry stool and hardness binding in the intestines and fullness and pain in the abdomen.

Analysis:

- Treats filth stagnating in the intestines because qì is unable to move it and the fluids are unable to moisten it.
- Appropriate for all symptoms of heat evil

spreading to the interior, forming glomus, fullness, dryness, repletion, and hardness.

- *Dà huáng* clears heat, *máng xiāo* moistens dryness, *hòu pò* moves qì, *zhǐ shí* attacks hardness.

麻黄加朮湯
Má Huáng Jiā Zhú Tāng

má huáng	麻黄	9g
guì zhī	桂枝	6g
gān cǎo	甘草	3g
bái zhú	白朮	12g
xìng rén	杏仁	70 pits

Indications: Dampness patients with generalized vexation and pain.

Analysis:

- Conditions of dampness (generalized pain) and heat (generalized vexation) in the exterior (absence of sweating).
- *Má Huáng Tāng* has the effect of promoting sweating and thereby dissipating the exterior.
- *Bái zhú* is added to supplement earth, engender liquid, and assist in eliminating dampness, because of the risk that great sweating damages yīn and resolves the exterior without removing dampness.

麻黄杏仁薏苡甘草湯
Má Huáng Xìng Rén Yì Yǐ Gān Cǎo Tāng

má huáng	麻黄	1.5g
xìng rén	杏仁	10 pits
yì yǐ rén	薏苡仁	1.5g
gān cǎo	甘草	3g

Indications: Wind dampness with generalized pain.

Analysis:

- Similar effect to *Má Huáng Jiā Zhú Tāng.*
- Pain all over the body indicates wind dampness brewing in the channels and network vessels.
- *Má huáng* dissipates wind-cold in the channels and network vessels.
- *Yì yǐ rén* sweeps away the dampness in the channels and network vessels.
- *Xìng rén* disinhibits lung qì.
- *Gān cǎo* supports the middle burner and amplifies the effect of *yì yǐ rén.*

防己黄芪湯
Fáng Jǐ Huáng Qí Tāng

fáng jǐ	防己	3g
gān cǎo	甘草	1.5g
bái zhú	白朮	2.25g
huáng qí	黄芪	3.75g

Indications: Wind-damp and wind water, with vexing pain in the joints, a floating pulse, heavy body, and sweating with aversion to wind.

Analysis:

- Treats exterior conditions (floating pulse) with wind damaging the interstices (aversion to wind) and dampness damaging the channels and network vessels (generalized heaviness).
- *Guì zhī* and *má huáng* effuse the exterior and drive out wind.
- *Huáng qí* penetrates the exterior and fills up emptiness.
- *Gān cǎo* and *bái zhú* supplement earth and overcome dampness.
- *Shēng jiāng* drives out wind and moves water with its warmth.
- *Fáng jǐ* penetrates everywhere, thereby leading the other medicinals to circulate throughout the entire body, freeing the outside and reaching the inside.

桂枝附子湯
Guì Zhī Fù Zǐ Tāng

guì zhī	桂枝	12g
shēng jiāng	生薑	9g
fù zǐ	附子	3 pcs
gān cǎo	甘草	6g
dà zǎo	大棗	12 pcs

Indications: Cold damage on the eighth or ninth day, when wind and dampness are struggling with each other. With vexing pain in the body and inability to turn to the side, no retching or thirst, and a pulse that is vacuous, floating, and rough.

Analysis:

- Treats wind-damp flowing into the channels and network vessels.
- *Guì zhī* dissipates wind in the exterior.
- *Fù zǐ* expels dampness from the channels.
- *Shēng jiāng, dà zǎo,* and *gān cǎo* move construction and defense and free the fluids.

白朮附子湯
Bái Zhú Fù Zǐ Tāng

bái zhú	白朮	6g
fù zǐ	附子	1.5 pcs
gān cǎo	甘草	3g
shēng jiāng	生薑	4.5g
dà zǎo	大棗	6 pcs

Indications: Wind vacuity, with heaviness and dizziness in the head and inability to taste food.

甘草附子湯
Gān Cǎo Fù Zǐ Tāng

gān cǎo	甘草	6g
bái zhú	白朮	6g
fù zǐ	附子	2 pcs
guì zhī	桂枝	12g

Indications: Wind-damp, with pain in the bones and joints, sweating with shortness of breath, inhibited urination, aversion to wind, and possibly mild swelling of the body.

Analysis:

- Treats both the interior and exterior.
- *Fù zǐ* expels dampness and warms the channels.
- *Guì zhī* drives out wind and harmonizes construction.
- *Bái zhú* gets rid of dampness and makes

defense replete.

- *Gān cǎo* assists all the other ingredients and moderates the dissipating effect because if the expelling action is too drastic, wind will be removed but dampness will stay.

白虎人參湯

Bái Hǔ Rén Shēn Tāng

zhī mǔ	知母	18g
shí gāo	石膏	48g
gān cǎo	甘草	6g
jīng mǐ	粳米	120ml
rén shēn	人參	9g

Indications: Tàiyáng diseases with relentless heat after sweating, with vexing thirst even though the patient is drinking water, possibly heat stroke in tàiyáng, sweating with aversion to cold, generalized heat and thirst.

Analysis:

- Sweating, aversion to wind, and generalized heat WITHOUT thirst is wind strike; generalized heat WITH thirst is heat stroke. Both are caused by cold damage and wind strike.
- Vacuity in the defense means insufficiency in the exterior, resulting in sweating, generalized heat, and aversion to cold.
- Always caused by ministerial fire damaging the lung.
- Can turn into malaria in shàoyīn or yángmíng.
- The sovereign of the formula is *shí gāo*, which treats fire heat in the triple burner, thereby clearing the lung and abating the fire therein.
- *Zhī mǔ* also drains heart fire from the lung and enriches the source of water.
- *Rén shēn* engenders liquid and boosts the damaged qì.
- *Jīng mǐ* and *gān cǎo* supplement earth to engender metal.

栝蒂散

Guā Dì Sǎn

guā dì 栝蒂 27 pcs

Indications: Floating *cùn* pulse with glomus in the chest, with abiding food in the upper stomach duct.

Analysis:

- Main formula for inducing vomiting.
- For conditions caused by cold, heat, damp turbidity, and phlegm-rheum brewing and binding in the chest.
- For conditions where treatment by promoting sweating or precipitation is ineffective.
- Formula uses sour and bitter emetics to free the upper burner and allow yáng qì to return.
- The extreme bitterness of *guā dì* eliminates repletion evil from the chest and stomach.
- Efficacy of the formula can be increased by taking it together with *xiāng chǐ* gruel to protect stomach qì.
- If no vomiting results, increase the dosage very slowly. As soon as vomiting occurs, stop immediately to prevent damage to original qì in the stomach.

百合知母湯
Bǎi Hé Zhī Mǔ Tāng

bǎi hé	百合	10 pcs
zhī mǔ	知母	9g

Indications: Hundred-Union disease after [erroneous treatment by] promoting sweating.
Analysis:

- Erroneous treatment of this condition by promoting sweating damages yīn, so we use this formula to safeguard yáng and thereby rescue yīn.
- Since the hundred vessels all face toward the lung, if they are all affected by disease, you can address the condition in the lung, which rules qì.
- *Bǎi hé* treats repletion of evil qì and supplements vacuity of right qì.
- *Zhī mǔ* enters lung metal to boost its source of water and frees the bladder in the lower body, causing the evil to be discharged in the urine.

百合滑石代赭石湯
Bǎi Hé Huá Shí Dài Zhě Shí Tāng

bǎi hé	百合	7 pcs
huá shí	滑石	9g
dài zhě shí	代赭石	1 pc the size of a pellet

Indications: Hundred-Union disease after [erroneous treatment by] precipitation.
Analysis:

- Erroneous precipitation in Hundred-Union disease invariably causes the heat to become entrapped, damaging yīn in the lower burner.
- *Bǎi hé* clears and supplements lung metal and moves the source of water.
- *Huá shí* guides heat qì and frees the water palace.
- *Dài zhě shí* prevents sweating and diarrhea.
- Hence the heat is discharged in the urine and the risk of burning yīn is avoided.

百合雞子黄湯
Bǎi Hé Jī Zǐ Huáng Tāng

bǎi hé	百合	7 pcs
egg yolk	雞子黄	1 pc

Indications: Hundred-Union disease after [erroneous treatment by] promoting vomiting.
Analysis:

- Erroneously treating Hundred-Union disease by inducing vomiting damages the fluids in the stomach.
- *Bǎi hé* enriches lung qì.
- Egg yolk quiets stomach qì.
- Since the stomach is the mother of the lung, quieting the stomach results in lung qì becoming harmonious.
- Both this and the previous formula exemplify the method of "treating yáng disease by rescuing yīn."

百合地黄湯

Bǎi Hé Dì Huáng Tāng

bǎi hé	百合	7 pcs
shēng dì huáng zhī	生地黄汁	200 ml

Indications: Hundred-Union disease that has not yet been treated by inducing vomiting, precipitation, or sweating.

Analysis:

- Outward appearance of the disease is similar to what it was at the onset.
- Caused by heat generated by chronic depression, damaging qì and blood.
- *Bǎi hé* is bitter and cold, clearing the heat from the qì aspect.
- *Dì huáng* juice is sweet and moistening, removing heat from the blood aspect.
- An example of "rescuing yīn by discharging heat" and "using yīn softness to transform yáng hardness."
- Heat being discharged in the stool manifests in lacquer-colored stool.

百合洗方

Bǎi Hé Xǐ Fāng

bǎi hé	百合	200 ml

Indications: Hundred-Union disease that has not been resolved in one month but has transformed to cause thirst.

Analysis:

- Here, evil heat has spread to the lung channel. Since the skin and body hair belong to the lung, washing the outside also frees the inside.
- In conjunction with this body wash, consume wheat cakes, to allow grain qì to transport the fluids.
- Salty fermented foods are contraindicated because salt consumes water and increases thirst.

栝蔞牡蠣散

Guā Lóu Mǔ Lì Sǎn

guā lóu gēn	栝蔞根
mǔ lì	牡蠣

Indications: Hundred-Union disease with unrelenting thirst.

Analysis:

- Unrelenting thirst indicates that internal yīn qì has not recovered in spite of treating the patient with the previous *Bǎi Hé Xǐ Fāng*.
- *Mǔ lì* subdues yáng and *guā lóu gēn* engenders liquids.

百合滑石散

Bǎi Hé Huá Shí Sǎn

bǎi hé	百合	3g
huá shí	滑石	9g

Indications: Hundred-Union disease that has transformed into heat effusion.

Analysis:

- Not an original symptom of Hundred-Union disease, heat effusion indicates that the internal heat is overflowing and oozing into the skin.
- *Bǎi hé* clears metal and drains fire, and leads

counterflow qì down from its high source.

- *Huá shí* abates heat in the interior and exterior and disinhibits urine.
- Using a powder (*sǎn*) to dissipate (*sàn*), this formula draws the heat out from the everywhere in the interior and exterior of the body to discharge it in the urine.

甘草瀉心湯
Gān Cǎo Xiè Xīn Tāng

gān cǎo	甘草	12g
huáng qín	黃芩	9g
gān jiāng	乾薑	9g
rén shēn	人參	9g
bàn xià	半夏	100ml
huáng lián	黃連	3g
dà zǎo	大棗	12 pcs

Indications: Erosion in the upper body that is a result of Fox-Creeper disease.
Analysis:

- Fox-Creeper is a disease related to worms, caused by damp-heat brewing in the stomach.
- The bitter and cold nature of *huáng qín* and *huáng lián*, in combination with the acrid and warm nature of *gān jiāng* and *bàn xià*, kills worms by harmonizing the stomach and transforming damp-heat.
- Fox-Creeper is always also rooted in vacuity of right qì, which is allowing worms to cause this disease.
- *Rén shēn*, *gān cǎo*, and *dà zǎo* supplement the center and hold on to right qì.

苦參湯
Kǔ Shēn Tāng

kǔ shēn	苦參	200ml

Indications: Fox-Creeper disease.
Analysis:

- The worms in Fox-Creeper disease are engendered after contracting wind-wood damp-heat qì. They die when they encounter bitterness and cold.
- *Kǔ shēn* is bitter and cold. Bitterness drains fire, cold abates heat. Its drying effect eliminates dampness.

雄黃熏法
Xióng Huáng Xūn Fǎ

xióng huáng	雄黃

Indications: Fox-Creeper disease.
Analysis:

- *Xióng huáng*, bitter and cold in nature, is able to get rid of damp-heat and kill worms.

赤小豆當歸散
Chì Xiǎo Dòu Dāng Guī Sǎn

chì xiǎo dòu	赤小豆	600ml
dāng guī	當歸	7.5g

Indications: Fox-Creeper disease causing blood in the stool.
Analysis:

- For damp-heat invading the genitals.

- *Chì xiǎo dòu* removes dampness, clears heat, and resolves toxin, treating disease in shàoyīn.
- *Dāng guī* leads heat down, nourishes blood, and disperses depression, treating disease in juéyīn.
- Taking the powder by drinking it with fermented grain-water harmonizes stomach qì, so that fire and earth and earth and wood are in harmony.

升麻鱉甲湯
Shēng Má Biē Jiǎ Tāng

shēng má	升麻	6g
dāng guī	當歸	3g
gān cǎo	甘草	3g
shǔ jiāo	蜀椒	3g
biē jiǎ	鱉甲	1 finger sized pc
xióng huáng	雄黃	1.5g

Indications: Yáng toxins, with a red face with marks that look like brocade lines, sore throat, and vomiting of pus and blood.

Analysis:

- Both yīn toxins and yáng toxins cause sore throat because the qì of toxic pestilence always enters through the nose and mouth.
- Yáng toxins, attaching themselves to the exterior, manifest in a red face with spots and lines and vomiting of pus and blood. Yīn toxins, hiding in the interior inside the exterior, manifest in a blue-green face and eyes and generalized pain as if having been beaten with a staff.
- *Shēng má* enters yángmíng and tàiyáng to upbear, clear, and drive out filth, eliminate the hundred evils, and resolve the hundred toxins, thereby controlling both yīn and yáng conditions of warm pestilence. But it only addresses the qì aspect.
- It is assisted here by *dāng guī*, which frees the blood in the network vessels; by *gān cǎo*, which resolves toxins in the network vessels; and by *biē jiǎ*, which guards and protects construction and the spirit.
- The fierce substances *shǔ jiāo* and *xióng huáng* attack toxins and outthrust the exterior.

鱉甲煎丸
Biē Jiǎ Jiān Wán

biē jiǎ	鱉甲	9g
wū shàn	烏扇	2.25g
huáng qín	黄芩	2.25g
chái hú	柴胡	4.5g
shǔ fù	鼠婦	2.25g
gān jiāng	乾薑	2.25g
dà huáng	大黃	2.25g
guì zhī	桂枝	2.25g
shí wéi	石韋	2.25g
hòu pò	厚朴	2.25g
zǐ wēi	紫葳	2.25g
bàn xià	半夏	3.75g
ē jiāo	阿膠	2.25g
sháo yào	芍藥	3.75g
mǔ dān pí	牡丹皮	3.75g
zhè chóng	䗪蟲	3.75g
tíng lì	葶藶	0.75g
rén shēn	人參	0.75g
qū mài	瞿麥	1.5g
fēng wō	蜂窠	3g
chì xiāo	赤硝	9g
qiāng láng	蜣螂	4.5g
táo rén	桃仁	1.5g

Indications: Mother of malaria.
Analysis:

- For conditions where chronic malaria has left construction and defense and has positioned itself in the viscera and bowels.
- The large amount of insect-based medicinals creates a fierce effect of moving qì and expelling evil from the blood.
- The sovereign here is therefore *biē jiǎ*, because of its guarding effect on the spirit, and because its efficacy in discharging from juéyīn and breaking concretions and accumulations is unmatched by any plant-based medicinals.
- *Ē jiāo* outthrusts the exterior and extinguishes wind. *Qiāng láng* is moving and upbearing by nature. The toxicity of *fēng wō* is able to lead substances downward and precipitate. *Zhè chóng* breaks blood. *Shǔ fù* penetrates the qì.
- *Tíng lì* discharges qì blockage, while *dà huáng* discharges blood blockage.
- *Chì xiāo* softens hardness, *táo rén* breaks binds, *wū shàn* downbears ministerial fire in juéyīn, *zǐ wēi* breaks bound blood in juéyīn.
- *Gān jiāng* harmonizes yáng and reduces cold, *huáng qín* harmonizes yīn and reduces heat.
- For harmonizing the interior and exterior, the formula contains *chái hú* and *guì zhī*. For balancing construction and defense, the formula contains *rén shēn*.
- *Sháo yào* and *hòu pò* outthrust from the origin to remove the evil from there. *Dān pí* enters yīn to remove the evil from there.
- *Shí wéi* opens up water in the upper burner, while *qū mài* flushes water from the lower burner.
- *Bàn xià* harmonizes the stomach and frees the flow of yīn and yáng.
- Stove ash is warm by nature and penetrates the qì. Clear liquor is slackening and penetrates the blood.
- All the medicinals here affect none other than the two channels of juéyīn and yángmíng.
- With the exception of *Shǔ Yù Wán*, no other formula in the *Jīn Guì Yào Lüè* contains this many ingredients.
- Both of these formulas treat conditions that are characterized by both vacuity of right and chronic presence of evil. Without gathering both blood-treating and qì-treating medicinals and without combining attack and supplementation, any treatment is pointless.

白虎加桂枝湯
Bái Hǔ Jiā Guì Zhī Tāng

zhī mǔ	知母	18g
shí gāo	石膏	48g
gān cǎo	甘草	6g
jīng mǐ	粳米	120ml
guì zhī	桂枝	9g

Indications: Warm malaria.
Analysis:

- The *Huáng Dì Nèi Jīng* discusses malaria that is caused by evil deep in the body, namely in the bones, characterized by heat effusion prior to aversion to cold.
- By contrast, this formula offers a treatment for malaria that is caused by evil that is shallow, namely in the heart, characterized by only heat and no cold.
- *Bái Hǔ Tāng* clears heat evil in the construction aspect, i.e., the heart.
- The addition of *guì zhī* leads *shí gāo* and *zhī*

mǔ up into the lung, discharging heat from the defense aspect as well.

蜀漆散
Shǔ Qī Sǎn

shǔ qī	蜀漆
yún mǔ	雲母
lóng gǔ	龍骨

Indications: Female malaria with a predominance of cold.

Analysis:

- *Shǔ qī* is upbearing by nature and gushes upward into the farthest reaches of the most obstinate phlegm.
- *Yún mǔ* is warming and scatters the fiercest strongholds of yīn evil.
- Because of the fierce gushing and draining effect of these medicinals, *lóng gǔ* is needed to secure the fluids. Being pure yáng in nature, it is helpful in dissipating evils that are lying latent in yīn.

牡蠣湯
Mǔ Lì Tāng

mǔ lì	牡蠣	12g
má huáng	麻黄	12g
gān cǎo	甘草	6g
shǔ qī	蜀漆	9g

Indications: Male malaria.

Analysis:

- Malaria with a predominance of cold signs is called male malaria. It is due to phlegm-rheum blocking the chest and obstructing the qì of heart yáng so it is unable to flow to the outside.
- *Mǔ lì* disperses binds.
- *Má huáng* dissipates cold and at the same time brings out yáng qì, allowing it to flow to the outside.

柴胡去半夏加栝蔞根湯
Chái Hú Qù Bàn Xià Jiā Guā Lóu Gēn Tāng

chái hú	柴胡	24g
rén shēn	人參	9g
huáng qín	黄芩	9g
gān cǎo	甘草	9g
guā lóu gēn	栝蔞根	12g
shēng jiāng	生薑	9g
dà zǎo	大棗	12 pcs

Indications: Treats malaria that erupts with thirst, as well as taxation malaria.

Analysis:

- In ordinary malaria with intermittent cold and heat, the evil erupts in shàoyáng, which is different from cold damage conditions where the evil erupts in shàoyáng.
- Shàoyáng malaria erupting with thirst is caused by an excess of wind-fire on the inside seizing the fluids.
- *Bàn xià* has been removed from the formula because it its slippery and disinhibiting by nature and therefore damages the yīn fluids.
- *Guā lóu gēn* engenders liquid and moistens dryness.

柴胡桂薑湯
Chái Hú Guì Jiāng Tāng

chái hú	柴胡	24g
guì zhī	桂枝	9g
gān jiāng	乾薑	6g
guā lóu gēn	栝蔞根	12g
huáng qín	黄芩	9g
gān cǎo	甘草	6g
mǔ lì	牡蠣	6g

Indications: Cold damage that has been treated first with sweating and then with precipitation. With fullness in the chest and rib-sides, mild binding, inhibited urination, thirst and no retching, sweating from the head, intermittent cold and heat, and vexation below the heart. Also treats malaria with predominant cold and only mild heat, or with only cold and no heat.

Analysis:

- If cold damage conditions have been treated with sweating and then with precipitation, the result is counterflow in the pivot of shàoyáng. The above symptoms show that the evil is unable to exit through the lower body, that fire qì is implicated in shàoyáng, and that the fluids in tàiyáng are steaming upward into the head.
- *Chái hú* harmonizes yáng in shàoyáng, hereby working in tandem with *huáng qín.*
- *Guì zhī* harmonizes yáng in tàiyáng, hereby working in tandem with *mǔ lì.*
- *Gān jiāng* harmonizes yáng in yángmíng, hereby working in tandem with *guā lóu gēn.*
- *Chái hú, guì zhī,* and *huáng qín* all revolve around the pivot of shàoyáng and outthurst the qì in tàiyáng.
- *Mǔ lì* opens up the qì in juéyīn, thereby resolving the binds in the chest and rib-sides.
- *Guā lóu gēn* draws fluids into the upper body and thereby stops vexing thirst.
- Because sweating and precipitation make center qì vacuous, the formula uses *gān cǎo* to regulate the center and harmonize yīn and yáng.
- The reason why the formula emphasizes *chái hú* among the yáng medicinals is that true malaria does not leave the hand shàoyáng channel.
- The formula emphasizes *guā lóu gēn* among the yīn medicinals because rescuing the fluids in this kind of malaria with yīn exhaustion is the most urgent priority.

侯氏黑散
Hóu Shì Hēi Sǎn

jú huā	菊花	30g
bái zhú	白朮	7.5g
fáng fēng	防風	7.5g
jié gěng	桔梗	6g
huáng qín	黄芩	3.75g
xì xīn	細辛	2.25g
gān jiāng	乾薑	2.25g
rén shēn	人參	2.25g
fú líng	茯苓	2.25g
dāng guī	當歸	2.25g
chuān xiōng	川芎	2.25g
mǔ lì	牡蠣	2.25g
fán shí	礬石	2.25g
guì zhī	桂枝	2.25g

Indications: Wind with vexation and heaviness in the four extremities, aversion to cold, and insufficiency in the heart.

Analysis:

- Spleen earth, when constrained by wind water, binds internally rather than spreading to the four extremities.
- Turbid qì is congesting the center of the chest, causing heart fire to brew internally so that the heat conversely transforms into cold.
- *Jú huā,* as the sovereign of the formula, resolves the smoldering heat below the heart.
- *Fáng fēng, guì zhī, xì xīn,* and *jié gěng* upbear and effuse the interstices.
- *Rén shēn, huáng qín,* and *bái zhú* dispel wind from the replete spleen.
- *Chuān xiōng* and *dāng guī* moisten dryness and extinguish fire.
- *Mǔ lì* and *fán shí* secure and astringe the intestines and stomach, preventing *rén shēn* and *bái zhú* from being too dissipating.
- Taking the formula with warm liquor makes the medicinals run into the exterior to open up any impediment.
- Consuming hot substances is contraindicated because *fán shí* when contracting heat, causes precipitation, which would prevent the medicinals from exerting their full strength.

風引湯

Fēng Yǐn Tāng

dà huáng	大黄	12g
gān jiāng	乾薑	12g
lóng gǔ	龍骨	12g
guì zhī	桂枝	9g
gān cǎo	甘草	6g
mǔ lì	牡蠣	6g
hán shuǐ shí	寒水石	18g
huá shí	滑石	18g
chì shí zhī	赤石脂	18g
bái shí zhī	白石脂	18g
zǐ shí yīng	紫石英	18g
shí gāo	石膏	18g

Indications: Heat paralysis and epilepsy. Also treats fright palpitations with tugging and pulling in infants.

Analysis:

- Wind engendered by fire heat invariably injures center earth.
- Paralysis means that wind wood complicated by phlegm has poured into the four extremities. Epilepsy means that wind-heat is harassing the channels.
- *Dà huáng* is the sovereign because it sweeps away the evils of wind, fire, heat, and dampness.
- *Gān jiāng* supplements by stopping flow.
- *Guì zhī* and *gān cǎo* moderate the force of the other medicinals.
- The minerals in this formula astringe to fill up the roadways: *Huá shí* and *shí gāo* clear metal to calm wood; *chì shí zhī* and *bái shí zhī* eliminate dampness and enlarge earth; *lóng gǔ* and *mǔ lì* restrain the confused and galloping essence spirit and *hún* and *pò* souls; *hán shuǐ shí* assists true yīn in the kidney; *zǐ shí yīng* supplements the vacuity of the heart spirit.

防己地黄湯
Fáng Jǐ Dì Huáng Tāng

fáng jǐ	防己	0.75g
gān cǎo	甘草	0.75g
guì zhī	桂枝	2.25g
fáng fēng	防風	2.25g

Indications: Wind strike that resembles mania, with no heat and a floating pulse.

Analysis:

- A formula that uses the clear juice produced by soaking fresh ingredients returns to yáng to dissipate evil. A formula that uses the thick juice produced by steaming ingredients with heat returns to yīn to supplement blood.
- In combination, this formula treats wind evil that has attached itself to the heart, causing epilepsy, fright, and mania. When we use the thick juice produced by steaming ingredients with heat, the formula returns to yīn to supplement blood.

頭風摩散
Tóu Fēng Mó Sǎn

dà fù zǐ	大附子	1 pc
yán	鹽	equal amounts

Indications: Great cold invading the brain and causing headache.

桂枝芍藥知母湯
Guì Zhī Sháo Yào Zhī Mǔ Tāng

guì zhī	桂枝	12g
sháo yào	芍藥	9g
gān cǎo	甘草	6g
má huáng	麻黃	6g
fù zǐ	附子	6g
bái zhú	白朮	12g
zhī mǔ	知母	12g
fáng fēng	防風	12g
shēng jiāng	生薑	15g

Indications: Pain in the extremities and joints, generalized lameness and emaciation, swelling in the feet as in desertion, dizziness in the head and shortness of breath, and a feeling of uncomfortable warmth and being on the verge of vomiting.

Analysis:

- This is *Guì Zhī Tāng* without *dà zǎo* but with *má huáng* added to free and harmonize the stagnation in the channels and network vessels.
- Adding *bái zhú* and *fáng fēng* extends spleen qì.
- *Sháo yào*, *fù zǐ*, and *zhī mǔ* balance yīn and yáng.
- The increased amount of *shēng jiāng* calms the retching and counterflow.

烏頭湯
Wū Tóu Tāng

má huáng	麻黃	9g
sháo yào	芍藥	9g

huáng qí	黃芪	9g
gān cǎo	甘草	9g
wū tóu	烏頭	5 pcs

Indications: Pain caused by joint-running, with inability to bend and stretch. Also treats the pain of leg qì.

Analysis:

- Proper treatment for cold-damp evil that causes joint-running.
- *Má huáng* and *wū tóu* are indispensable in removing cold-damp.
- Because the disease is in the joints and not in the skin and body hair, we cannot dissipate it by sweating.
- The supplementing effect of *huáng qí*, calming effect of *bái sháo*, and moderating effect of *gān cǎo* are necessary to restrain the two harsh medicinals, so that the formula can enter deeply to get rid of the evil.

礬石湯

Fán Shí Tāng

fán shí	礬石	6g

Indications: Leg qì surging against the heart.

Analysis:

- Leg qì means that dampness has damaged the lower body and qì is surging into the upper body.
- *Fán shí*, being sour and astringent, is drying and thereby able to gather dampness and resolve toxin.

續命湯

Xù Mìng Tāng

má huáng	麻黃	9g
guì zhī	桂枝	9g
rén shēn	人參	9g
gān cǎo	甘草	9g
gān jiāng	乾薑	9g
shí gāo	石膏	9g
dāng guī	當歸	9g
chuān xiōng	川芎	4.5g
xìng rén	杏仁	40 pits

Indications: Wind strike with prickly heat, with inability to contract the body and hold it together, inability to speak, veiling and confusion so that the patient doesn't know the location of the pain, possibly hypertonicity and inability to turn to the side, possibly a hidden pulse with inability to rest, cough with counterflow qì ascent, and puffy swelling in the face and eyes.

Analysis:

- Main formula for treating wind strike conditions.
- In treatment, distinguish carefully between vacuity conditions (contracted due to inappropriate drink and diet, bedroom taxation, and the seven emotions) and repletion conditions (wind, cold, summerheat, and dampness).
- Addresses repletion evil in construction and defense by dispelling wind and penetrating the exterior, calming the interior and resisting on the exterior, and circulating all over the upper and lower body.
- *Má huáng, guì zhī, gān jiāng, xìng rén, shí gāo*, and *gān cǎo* disperse wind evil in the fleshy exterior and regulate the heat brewing

in the interior.

- *Dāng guī* harmonizes blood, *rén shēn* boosts qì, *chuān xiōng* moves blood, dissipates wind, leads the various medicinals into the sinews and bones, frees the channels and network vessels, and outthrusts the evil from the inside through the fleshy exterior.

三黃湯

Sān Huáng Tāng

má huáng	麻黃	3.75g
dú huó	獨活	3g
xì xīn	細辛	1.5g
huáng qí	黃芪	1.5g
huáng qín	黃芩	2.25g

Indications: Wind strike with hypertension and pain, with hemilateral paralysis, muteness, vexing heat and derangement in the heart, aversion to cold, no desire for food and drink. Also treats bandit wind and *wěi tuǐ* wind.[1]

Analysis:

- *Má huáng* and *huáng qí* enter tàiyīn to perfuse yáng, effuse the exterior, and drive out evil from the spleen.
- *Xì xīn* and *dú huó* enter the kidney and penetrate the sinews and bones, to dissipate evil from the kidney.
- *Huáng qín* clears internal heat to stop vexation.
- For vexing heat in the heart that *huáng qín* is unable to expel, add *dà huáng* to lead it down and discharge it by means of precipitation.
- Adding *zhǐ shí, rén shēn, mǔ lì*, and *guā lóu gēn* either treats effulgent qì or assists the root origin.
- The addition of *fù zǐ* supports the steaming dissipating action of *má huáng*. This combination is similar to *Má Huáng Fù Zǐ Xì Xīn Tāng*.

朮附湯

Zhú Fù Tāng

bái zhú	白朮	6g
fù zǐ	附子	1.5 pcs
gān cǎo	甘草	3g

Indications: Relaxes the muscles, supplements the center, and boosts essence qì. Treats wind vacuity with heaviness and dizziness in the head. Also treats wind and dampness struggling and causing reversal, with sudden fulminant heart pain, a slight pulse and weak qì, generalized vexation and pain, generalized cold with spontaneous sweating, no retching and no thirst, uninhibited urination, and hard stools.

Analysis:

- No wind medicinals among the formula ingredients!
- ***Fù zǐ*** warms the water viscus, and *bái zhú* and *gān cǎo* warm the earth viscus.
- When water and earth are both warm, the qì of turbid yīn all rushes into the lower body and all the symptoms disappear.

1. An ancient disease in the category of wind strike, also written as 猥退風 and described as characterized by unilateral paralysis of the extremities and muteness. See *Qiān Jīn Fāng*, vol. 8.

八味丸
Bā Wèi Wán

gān dì huáng	乾地黃	24g
shān zhū yú	山茱萸	12g
shǔ yù	薯蕷	12g
zé xiè	澤瀉	9g
fú líng	茯苓	9g
mǔ dān pí	牡丹皮	9g
guì zhī	桂枝	3g
fù zǐ	附子	3g

Indications: See below for *Bā Wèi Shèn Qì Wán.*

越婢加朮湯
Yuè Bì Jiā Zhú Tāng

má huáng	麻黃	18g
shí gāo	石膏	24g
gān cǎo	甘草	6g
shēng jiāng	生薑	9g
bái zhú	白朮	12g
dà zǎo	大棗	12 pcs

Indications: Water in the interior, with yellow coloration and swelling all over the body, in the face, and eyes, a sunken pulse, and inhibited urination. Also treats extreme heat in the interior with openness of the interstices and severe sweating, as well as pestilential wind qì with weakness in the lower burner and feet.

Analysis:

- This is *Yuè Bì Tāng* with the addition of *bái zhú.*
- Since *Yuè Bì Tāng* can disperse generalized swelling, it can also dissipate internally smoldering heat.
- *Bái zhú* is able to support the spleen and thereby control water. Hence it can also secure the interstices and check sweating.

黃芪桂枝五物湯
Huáng Qí Guì Zhī Wǔ Wù Tāng

huáng qí	黃芪	9g
sháo yào	芍藥	9g
guì zhī	桂枝	9g
shēng jiāng	生薑	18g
dà zǎo	大棗	12 pcs

Indications: Blood impediment with dual debilitation of yīn and yáng, with a pulse that is faint at *cùn kǒu* and above *guān* and slightly tight at *chǐ*, generalized numbness, and an appearance like wind impediment. Also treats wind *féi* disablement.

Analysis:

- Wind evil in one half of the body, when compounded by vacuity in construction and defense, enters deep into the body and becomes chronic, forming signs like hemilateral withering and paralysis.
- When compounded by repletion in construction and defense, it enters the shallow areas and remains for a shorter period, forming signs like hemilateral pain and wind impediment.
- Use this formula in vacuity patterns to supplement what is lacking.
- The sovereign is *huáng qí,* which supplements defense.
- The ministers *guì zhī* and *sháo yào* supplement construction.

- The assistants *gān jiāng* and *dà zǎo* diffuse the qì, thereby preventing qì from stagnating and expelling impediment.
- This is a modification of *Xiǎo Jiàn Zhōng Tāng*.

桂枝龍骨牡蠣湯
Guì Zhī Lóng Gǔ Mǔ Lì Tāng

guì zhī	桂枝	9g
sháo yào	芍藥	9g
shēng jiāng	生薑	9g
gān cǎo	甘草	6g
dà zǎo	大棗	12 pcs
lóng gǔ	龍骨	9g
mǔ lì	牡蠣	9g

Indications: Seminal loss in men, with tension in the lesser abdomen, cold in the penis, dizzy vision and hair loss, and a pulse that is extremely vacuous, scallion-stalk, and slow. Also treats dreams of intercourse [with ghosts] in women.

Analysis:

- To address symptoms on the outside of the body, *Guì Zhī Tāng* is able to resolve the flesh and remove evil qì. To address symptoms on the inside, it is able to supplement vacuity and balance yīn and yáng.
- The combination of *lóng gǔ*, being the remains from the dragon moulting, and *mǔ lì*, being the bound quintessence of the ocean, adds the action of submerging yáng and astringing essence, to treat seminal loss and sexual dreams and thereby control the risk of the essence and spirit floating astray.

天雄散
Tiān Xióng Sǎn

tiān xióng	天雄	9g
bái zhú	白朮	24g
guì zhī	桂枝	18g
lóng gǔ	龍骨	9g

Indications: Insecurity of yīn essence.

Analysis:

- Formula is strongly warming and supplementing, while also settling and promoting absorption.
- *Bái zhú* enters the spleen to promote the intake of grain, since grain engenders essence.
- *Guì zhī* enters the gallbladder to transform qì since qì also engenders essence.
- *Lóng gǔ* contains essence and returns it to the kidney.
- Exemplifies the rule from the *Huáng Dì Nèi Jīng*: "When the kidney is injured, boost the essence."
- If *tiān xióng* is difficult to find, you can substitue *fù zǐ*.

小建中湯
Xiǎo Jiàn Zhōng Tāng

guì zhī	桂枝	9g
gān cǎo	甘草	6g
dà zǎo	大棗	12 pcs
sháo yào	芍藥	18g
shēng jiāng	生薑	9g
jiāo yí	膠飴	200ml

Indications: Unresolved cold damage in the exterior, with a rough yáng pulse and stringlike yīn pulse, vexation and palpitations in the heart, and tension and pain in the abdomen. Also treats vacuity taxation with abdominal urgency, with palpitations and nosebleed and abdominal pain. Also treats seminal loss during dreaming, with soreness in the four extremities, vexing heat in the hands and feet, and dry throat and mouth.

Analysis:

- This formula is *Guì Zhī Tāng* with double the amount of *sháo yào* and the addition of malt sugar.
- Palpitations mean yáng vacuity; vexation means yīn vacuity. Cold qì entering the yáng network vessels makes the yáng pulse rough; entering the yīn network vessels, it makes the yīn pulse stringlike.
- Insufficiency in construction and defense means vacuity in the exterior. Wind entering earth means tension in the interior.
- Even though the center is vacuous, the exterior is not yet harmonized. Therefore do not yet supplement strongly!
- With bitterness and sourness, the sovereign *sháo yào* boosts yīn and is able to drain wood from within earth.
- The warmth of the ministers malt sugar and *gān cǎo* supplements the spleen and nourishes the stomach.
- The acrid heat of *guì zhī* is used to support yáng and remove cold water.
- The acrid warmth of *shēng jiāng* and *dà zǎo*, as the envoys, is able to dissipate yáng qì.
- Take the formula warm to cause sweating.
- The emphasis of the formula is on treating the vacuity in the center, not the cold damage in the exterior.
- Because of the sweetness, this formula is contraindicated in patients suffering from retching and for alcoholics.

黄芪建中湯

Huáng Qí Jiàn Zhōng Tāng

huáng qí	黄芪	4.5g
guì zhī	桂枝	9g
gān cǎo	甘草	6g
dà zǎo	大棗	12 pcs
sháo yào	芍藥	18g
shēng jiāng	生薑	9g
jiāo yí	膠飴	200 ml

Indications: Vacuity taxation with abdominal urgency and the various forms of insufficiency.

Analysis:

- This is with the addition of *huáng qí*.
- *Xiǎo Jiàn Zhōng Tāng* uses sweetness and warmth to support the spleen and stomach, addressing the insufficiency.
- The addition of *huáng qí*, which greatly boosts original qì, bolsters its effect.
- Because of the sticky nature of *huáng qí*, which can stagnate in the stomach causing shortness of breath and fullness in the chest, we add *shēng jiāng* to move it.
- Fullness in the abdomen means stagnation in the intestines. Remove *dà zǎo* and add *fú líng*.
- For patients with lung vacuity and weakness in the qì aspect, add *bàn xià*.

八味腎氣丸
Bā Wèi Shèn Qì Wán

gān dì huáng	乾地黃	24g
shān yào	山藥	12g
shān zhū yú	山茱萸	12g
zé xiè	澤瀉	9g
mǔ dān pí	牡丹皮	9g
fú líng	茯苓	9g
guì zhī	桂枝	3g
fù zǐ	附子	3g

Indications: Vacuity taxation with lumbar pain. Also treats dispersion-thirst with increased urination in men and shifted bladder with inability to urinate in women.

Analysis:

- *Gan dì huáng* and *shān yào* enrich kidney yīn.
- *Shān zhū yú* and *fù zǐ* strengthen kidney yáng.
- *Guì zhī* transforms visceral qì.
- *Fú líng* promotes movement in the waterways.
- *Dān pí* and *zé xiè* eliminate toxic matter from within the blood and support the kidney in its task of qì transformation. Hence we reduce the increased urination and free the blockage.

薯蕷丸
Shǔ Yù Wán

shǔ yù	薯蕷	22.5g
rén shēn	人參	5.25g
bái zhú	白朮	4.5g
fú líng	茯苓	3.75g
gān cǎo	甘草	15g
dāng guī	當歸	7.5g
sháo yào	芍藥	4.5g
chuān xiōng	川芎	4.5g
gān dì huáng	乾地黃	7.5g
mài mén dōng	麥門冬	4.5g
ē jiāo	阿膠	5.25g
gān jiāng	乾薑	2.25g
dà zǎo	大棗	100 pcs
jié gěng	桔梗	3.75g
xìng rén	杏仁	4.5g
guì zhī	桂枝	7.5g
fáng fēng	防風	4.5g
shén qū	神曲	7.5g
chái hú	柴胡	3.75g
bái liǎn	白蘞	1.5g
dòu huáng juǎn	豆黃卷	7.5g

Indications: Vacuity taxation and all forms of insufficiency. Also treats the hundred diseases of wind qì.

Analysis:

- Original qì is located in the lung, original yáng in the kidney. Extreme deprivation means that the patient must rely on the acquired grain qì to boost it.
- This formula is ruled by *shǔ yù,* which specializes in regulating the spleen and stomach and supporting injury both in the upper and lower body.
- *Rén shēn, bái zhú, fú líng, gān jiāng, dòu huáng juǎn, dà zǎo, shén qū,* and *gān cǎo* eliminate dampness and boost qì.
- *Dāng guī, chuān xiōng, sháo yào, dì huáng, mài mén dōng,* and *ē jiāo* nourish blood and enrich yīn.
- *Chái hú, guì zhī,* and *fáng fēng* drive out evil

and dissipate heat.

- *Xìng rén, jié gěng,* and *bái liǎn* open up the depressed qì in the lower body.

酸棗仁湯
Suān Zǎo Rén Tāng

suān zǎo rén	酸棗仁	400ml
gān cǎo	甘草	3g
zhī mǔ	知母	6g
fú líng	茯苓	6g
chuān xiōng	川芎	3g

Indications: Vacuity taxation with insomnia. Also treats night sweating.

Analysis:

- Vacuity taxation means insufficiency of true yīn. Vacuity fire ascending into the brain causes sleeplessness because of the heat.
- The sour and bitter flavor of the sovereign *suān zǎo rén* has the effect of draining depressed heat from the brain.
- The acridity of *chuān xiōng* scurries upward to outthrust the heat.
- *Zhī mǔ* cools and *gān cǎo* harmonizes.
- Since dampness can stagnate instead of moving into the lower body, we use *fú líng* to sweep free its path and remove all obstacles.
- Nightsweats are caused by heat in the stomach and vacuity in the liver.
- *Zhī mǔ* cools the stomach and *gān cǎo* harmonizes it.
- *Suān zǎo rén* and *chuān xiōng* course the liver and control liver vacuity.

大黄䗪蟲丸
Dà Huáng Zhè Chóng Wán

dà huáng	大黃	7.5g
huáng qín	黃芩	6g
gān cǎo	甘草	9g
táo rén	桃仁	200ml
xìng rén	杏仁	200ml
sháo yào	芍藥	12g
gān qī	乾漆	3g
méng chóng	虻蟲	200ml
gān dì huáng	乾地黃	30g
shuǐ zhì	水蛭	100 pcs
qí cáo	蠐螬	100 pcs
zhè chóng	䗪蟲	100ml

Indications: The five taxations, with extreme vacuity, marked emaciation, abdominal fullness, and inability to drink and eat. Also treats damage from food, from worrying, from drink, from sexual intercourse, from hunger, from taxation, and damage to qì in the channels and network vessels and construction and defense, with internal presence of dry blood, scaly dry skin, and darkness in both eyes.

Analysis:

- Chronic steaming of vacuity fire from the five taxations causes the formation of dry blood when it binds in the channels and network vessels.
- Stagnation means that newly engendered blood is unable to flow freely and reach everywhere, causing daily worsening emaciation that eventually leads do death.
- The formula's sovereign *dà huáng* diffuses stagnation in the stomach network vessels and moistens dryness.
- The assistant *huáng qín* clears lung defense.

- *Xìng rén* moistens heart construction, *táo rén* supplements liver vacuity, *gān dì huáng* enriches kidney dryness.
- With its rash and flying nature, *gān qī* breaks static blood in the spleen, stomach, and joints. Being upbearing, *méng chóng* enters the yáng aspect to break up blood while *shuǐ zhì*, being downbearing, enters the yīn aspect to dispel stasis. *Qí cáo* removes hard blood from below both rib-sides while *zhè chóng* breaks hardness, frees the network vessels, and moves yáng.
- *Sháo yào* and *gān cǎo* support the spleen and stomach and resolve the toxicity of the other medicinals.

炙甘草湯
Zhì Gān Cǎo Tāng

gān cǎo	甘草	12g
guì zhī	桂枝	9g
shēng jiāng	生薑	9g
mài mén dōng	麥門冬	100ml
má rén	麻仁	100ml
rén shēn	人參	6g
ē jiāo	阿膠	6g
dà zǎo	大棗	30 pcs
dì huáng	地黃	48g

Indications: Cold damage with a bound and regularly interrupted pulse, heart stirring and palpitations, lung wilting with profuse drooling and salivating, an uncomfortably warm and flustered feeling in the heart, vacuity taxation and insufficiency, and oppression after sweating.

Analysis:

- For a weak pulse, Zhāng Zhòngjǐng recommends adding *sháo yào* to this formula to boost yīn in yīn vacuity or adding *guì zhī* to free yáng in yáng vacuity. In severe cases, add *rén shēn* to engender the pulse.
- The discomfort in the heart indicates insufficiency of heart blood, which causes heart fire to flare upward and eventually overcome metal, causing lung wilting.
- *Dì huáng* is the sovereign and *mài mén dōng* as the minister, to drastically supplement true yīn.
- *Rén shēn* and *guì zhī* are necessary to free the yáng vessels; *shēng jiāng* and *dà zǎo* to harmonize construction and defense; *ē jiāo* to supplement blood; *má rén* to moisten binding in the intestines and stomach; and *gān cǎo* to moderate the effect of the formula and prevent rapid precipitation.
- By simmering the ingredients in clear liquor, you accelerate movement in the upper body.
- This formula enriches fluids, moistens dryness, nourishes yīn, and ties together yáng.

肘後獺肝散
Tǎ Gān Sǎn

tǎ gān	獺肝	one liver

Indications: Vacuity taxation, corpse infixation, and demon infixation.

Analysis:

- Vacuity infixation is always characterized by an involvement of worms.
- Otter liver is warm by nature and has the ability to kill worms. Hence it is an important medicine for treating patterns like vacuity taxation corpse infixation.

甘草乾薑湯
Gān Cǎo Gān Jiāng Tāng

gān cǎo	甘草	12g
gān jiāng	乾薑	6g

Indications: Tàiyáng patterns that have been erroneously treated by promoting sweating, with yáng vacuity in the stomach, vomiting with counterflow and dry throat, and vexing dryness and reversal. Also treats lung wilting with drool foaming at the mouth but no cough and no thirst, dizziness in the head, and enuresis and frequent urination.

Analysis:

- Treats vacuity in the stomach that is complicated by cold.
- Even though lung wilting is a heat pattern, it is related to vacuity due to collapse of the fluids. If treated with a bitter and cold formula, the bitterness can be transformed by fire to increase the heat, and the cold in the formula ingredients might not get absorbed.
- This formula is ruled by the great sweetness of *gān cǎo* and the out-thrusting effect of blast-fried *gān jiāng*, using its acrid and warm nature in a bitter and warm application.
- This formula exemplifies the method of "using sweetness and warmth to eliminate great heat," in combination with the method of quickening.
- Even though there is no reversal counterflow, but only a sunken pulse, fear of cold, and retching and vomiting and diarrhea, the indications for this formula belong to the *Sì Nì Tāng* pattern.

射乾麻黄湯
Shè Gān Má Huáng Tāng

shè gān	射乾	9g
má huáng	麻黄	12g
shēng jiāng	生薑	12g
xì xīn	細辛	9g
zǐ wǎn	紫菀	9g
kuǎn dōng huā	款冬花	9g
dà zǎo	大棗	7 pcs
bàn xià	半夏	100ml
wǔ wèi zǐ	五味子	100ml

Indications: Water rheum damaging the lung, with cough with qì ascent and sounds like a frog in the throat.

Analysis:

- Cold rheum from the lung that ascends into the throat irritates the inhaled and exhaled breath, hence causing a frog-like sound.
- In the formula, *shè gān, zǐ wǎn,* and *kuǎn dōng huā* disinhibit lung qì.
- *Má huáng, xì xīn,* and *shēng jiāng* dissipate evil qì.
- *Bàn xià* downbears counterflow qì.
- *Dà zǎo,* which quiets the center, and *wǔ wèi zǐ,* which constrains the lung, are included because there is a risk that the dissipating medicinals could harm right qì.

皂莢丸
Zào Jiá Wán

zào jiá	皂莢	24g

Indications: Lung welling-abscess at the onset, with cough with counterflow and qì ascent, and turbid spittle.

Analysis:

- Treats phlegm accumulating in the chest and binding instead of resolving, possibly with cough, panting, glomus, or welling-abscess.
- *Zào jiá* opens the congestion and sweeps away the filth.
- Adding *dà zǎo* paste calms stomach qì, so that the formula still nourishes right qì while expelling evil.
- This is the ancestor of formulas like *Qiān Mín Tāng* 千緡湯.

厚朴麻黄湯
Hòu Pò Má Huáng Tāng

hòu pò	厚朴	15g
má huáng	麻黄	12g
shí gāo	石膏	1 pc the size of a chicken egg
xìng rén	杏仁	100ml
bàn xià	半夏	100ml
gān jiāng	乾薑	6g
xì xīn	細辛	6g
xiǎo mài	小麥	200ml
wǔ wèi zǐ	五味子	100ml

Indications: Cough with a floating pulse, ascent of qì with fullness in the chest and inhibition in the throat, and frog-like sounds.

Analysis:

- Cough with a floating pulse indicates the presence of rheum on the inside that is being stirred by evil in the exterior. Encroaching on the upper body, it causes occlusion of yáng in the heart and lung.
- *Hòu pò* and *má huáng* both perfuse the yáng of the upper burner and downbear the rheum that has ascended counterflow, thereby widening the chest and opening the occlusion.
- *Xìng rén* frees lung qì and assists *má huáng* in resolving the exterior and removing the evil.
- *Gān jiāng, wǔ wèi zǐ, bàn xià,* and *xì xīn* all transform phlegm and sweep away the rheum.
- *Xiǎo mài* protects the heart ruler. First boiling it separately causes it to supplement the heart and nourish the fluids, while also leading the other medicinals from the lower body into the upper body.
- Without heavy substances, internal rheum is hard to calm, so the formula uses *shí gāo* to precipitate water rheum, addressing the issue of counterflow ascent.

澤漆湯
Zé Qī Tāng

bàn xià	半夏	100ml
zé qī	澤漆	600ml
zǐ shēn	紫參	15g
shēng jiāng	生薑	15g
bái qián	白前	15g
gān cǎo	甘草	9g
huáng qín	黄芩	9g

rén shēn	人參	9g
guì zhī	桂枝	9g

Indications: Rheum with a sunken pulse. Also treats ascent of qì with inhibition in the throat.

Analysis:

- Cough with a sunken pulse means that the disease is located in the interior in tàiyáng, as well as in the exterior in shàoyīn. Evil in tàiyáng means that the skin and body hair are damaged, which necessarily affects the lung, preventing it from engendering water. In addition, the pivot of shàoyīn moves counterflow in the lower body, so that the flow in the water ways is stopped. Hence internal rheum runs counterflow into the upper body, causing cough.
- Being bitter and cold, the sovereign *zé qī* invigorates the kidney and disinhibits water, hence checking the cough. It leads the other medicinals into the kidney and fills up kidney qì.
- *Bái qián* perfuses lung qì, *huáng qín* drains lung heat, *rén shēn* supplements lung vacuity, *gān cǎo* calms the spleen, *zǐ wǎn* opens up bindings, *guì zhī* transforms the bladder, *bàn xià* downbears counterflow, and *shēng jiāng* sweeps away the rheum.

麥門冬湯
Mài Mén Dōng Tāng

mài mén dōng	麥門冬	1,400ml
bàn xià	半夏	200ml
rén shēn	人參	6g
gān cǎo	甘草	6g
jīng mǐ	粳米	60ml
dà zǎo	大棗	12 pcs

Indications: Fire counterflow with ascent of qì and inhibition in the throat.

Analysis:

- This formula is a modification of *Bái Hǔ Jiā Rén Shēn Tāng*, with *shí gāo* and *zhī mǔ* removed and *mài mén dōng, bàn xià*, and *dà zǎo* added, to treat conditions related to dryness of the fluids in the stomach and vacuity fire flaming upward.
- If we interpret the symptoms simplistically only as a struggle between fire and heat and fail to recognize the need to supplement right qì and engender fluids, and thus treat this indication erroneously with medicinals that downbear fire and with cold medicinals, the result will be that fire rises even more and that the heat turns into blazing. This is not only pointless, but even harmful!
- In lung disease, the presence of stomach qì means life and the absence of stomach qì means death, because stomach qì is the mother qì of the lung!
- *Mài mén dōng, rén shēn, gān cǎo, dà zǎo,* and *jīng mǐ* strongly supplement center qì to engender fluids.
- The addition of *bàn xià*, being acrid and warm, has the effect of opening up the stomach, moving fluids, and moistening the lung.

葶藶大棗瀉肺湯
Tíng Lì Dà Zǎo Xiè Fèi Tāng

tíng lì	葶藶	1 pellet the size of a chicken egg
dà zǎo	大棗	12 pcs

Indications: Welling-abscess in the lung, with panting and inability to lie down, fullness and distention in the chest, puffy swelling all over the body, in the face, and in the eyes, nasal congestion with clear snivel, inability to discern fragrant or foul smells and sour or acrid flavors, cough with counterflow ascent of qì, panting and rasping sounds with distress and congestion, as well as propping rheum with inability to breathe.

Analysis:

- This formula merely uses the bitter and cold nature of *tíng lì* to enter the lung and discharge the qì blockage, supported by the sweet warmth of *dà zǎo* to supplement spleen earth and harmonize the force of the medicine.

桔梗湯
Jié Gěng Tāng

jié gěng	桔梗	3g
gān cǎo	甘草	6g

Indications: Shàoyīn throat pain and welling-abscess in the lung, with cough, fullness, and ejection of pus, wind-heat in the viscus of the heart causing cough, a block-like obstruction inside the throat, and in serious cases swelling and impediment in the throat.

Analysis:

- This formula ingeniously combines just two ingredients, *jié gěng* for opening and *gān cǎo* for clearing, thereby dispersing any fire qì in the top of the throat and above the lung.

越婢加半夏湯
Yuè Bì Jiā Bàn Xià Tāng

má huáng	麻黃	18g
shí gāo	石膏	24g
shēng jiāng	生薑	9g
dà zǎo	大棗	12 pcs
gān cǎo	甘草	6g
bàn xià	半夏	100ml

Indications: Lung distention with rheum and ascent of qì, manifesting with panting, eyes that look like they are about to fall out, and a floating large pulse.

Analysis:

- A treatment for lung distention, which is caused by wind and water struggling, and heat qì soaring upward, steaming the florid canopy, and running into the empty interstices.
- The addition of *bàn xià* to the formula has the effect of opening the pathways that are blocked by phlegm stagnation.
- In this combination, *shí gāo* is able to rely on the acrid heat to drive out phlegm and *bàn xià* is able to rely on the acrid coolness to clear heat.

小青龍加石膏湯
Xiǎo Qīng Lóng Jiā Shí Gāo Tāng

má huáng	麻黃	9g
sháo yào	芍藥	9g
guì zhī	桂枝	9g
xì xīn	細辛	9g
gān cǎo	甘草	9g

gān jiāng	乾薑	9g
wǔ wèi zǐ	五味子	100ml
bàn xià	半夏	100ml
shí gāo	石膏	6g

Indications: Lung distention with cough and ascent of qì, vexation, agitation, and panting, presence of water qì below the heart, and a floating pulse.

Analysis:

- In comparison with the above formula *Yuè Bì Jiā Bàn Xià Tāng*, which addresses external evil with distention and tonicity in the lung, the present formula addresses external evil that is complicated by internal heat, thus manifesting also with vexation and agitation in the lung. Both formulas are preventative treatments for lung qì, to avoid the formation of welling-abscess or wilting.
- Lung distention, rheum, and ascent of qì mean that internal evil and external rheum are struggling with each other.
- While sweating and diffusion are appropriate treatments, you must guard against further damage to liquid by the heat, hence the additional amount of *shí gāo*.
- Water below the heart requires the use of warm medicinals to open and remove it, hence we use *Xiǎo Qīng Lóng Jiā Shí Gāo Tāng*, which is both cold and warm.

生薑甘草湯

Shēng Jiāng Gān Cǎo Tāng

shēng jiāng	生薑	15g
rén shēn	人參	9g
gān cǎo	甘草	12g
dà zǎo	大棗	15 pcs

Indications: Lung wilting, with cough with drooling of foamy spittle, dryness in the throat, and thirst.

Analysis:

- *Shēng jiāng* is the sovereign, breaking yīn and moving yáng, to steam the fluids and enrich the upper body.
- The assistant *rén shēn* enters tàiyīn which arouses yáng in the spleen and fosters yīn in the lung.
- *Gān cǎo* and *dà zǎo* aid by supporting the beginning of life and making earth exuberant, so that it can engender metal to the point where it can restrain water.

桂枝去芍藥加皂莢湯

Guì Zhī Qù Sháo Yào Jiā Zào Jiá Tāng

guì zhī	桂枝	9g
shēng jiāng	生薑	9g
gān cǎo	甘草	9g
dà zǎo	大棗	12 pcs
zào jiá	皂莢	1 pc

Indications: Lung welling-abscess with vomiting of foamy drool at the onset and presence of evil in the exterior.

Analysis:

- In this formula, acrid and warm *guì zhī* and *shēng jiāng* are the sovereigns, moving yáng and dispersing yīn.
- They are assisted by the sweet moistening action of *dà zǎo* and *gān cǎo*, supplementing yīn and engendering fluids.
- For opening blockages and sweeping away filth to clean away the foamy drool, *zào jiá* is particularly well-suited.

桔梗白散

Jié Gěng Bái Sǎn

jié gěng	桔梗	2.25g
bèi mǔ	貝母	2.25g
bā dòu	巴豆	0.75g

Indications: Tàiyáng disease with cold repletion binding in the chest. Also treats lung welling-abscess.

Analysis:

- The acrid heat of *bā dòu* is able to dissipate cold repletion and break up water rheum.
- *Bèi mǔ* opens the chest bind.
- *Jié gěng* opens lung qì.
- Processing these medicinals into a powder increases the dissipating effect.
- Taking the powder with hot gruel reinforces the heat of *bā dòu* and thereby causes movement. Taking it with cold gruel restrains the heat of *bā dòu* and thereby stops movement. Taking the powder with gruel instead of water allows grain qì to protect stomach qì.

葦莖湯

Wěi Jīng Tāng

wěi jīng	葦莖	400ml
yì yǐ rén	薏苡仁	100ml
táo rén	桃仁	50 pcs
guā bàn	栝瓣	100ml

Indications: Lung welling-abscess, manifesting in cough with mild heat, vexation and fullness, and dry scaly skin in the middle of the chest.

Analysis:

- Treats damp-heat binding in the lung, obstructing the flow of qì and blood, and causing welling-abscess.
- *Wěi jīng* resolves the heat binding in the qì aspect.
- *Táo rén* drains the heat binding in the blood aspect.
- *Yì yǐ rén* disinhibits dampness and clears the source of binding heat.
- *Guā bàn* expels depression and opens the pathways of binding heat.
- The second dose should result in vomiting of a pus-like substance, which means that the force of the medicinals has moved to break the welling-abscess.

奔豚湯

Bēn Tún Tāng

gān cǎo	甘草	6g
dāng guī	當歸	6g
chuān xiōng	川芎	6g
huáng qín	黃芩	6g
sháo yào	芍藥	6g
bàn xià	半夏	12g
shēng jiāng	生薑	12g
shēng gé	生葛	15g
gān lǐ gēn bái pí	甘李根白皮	200ml

Indications: Running piglet surging up into the chest, with cold and heat and abdominal pain.

Analysis:

- Any ascent or descent of qì, regardless of whether it is right or evil qì, always starts from shàoyáng, which is the road of yīn and yáng.

- Struggle between yīn and yáng means abdominal pain; upbearing qì means heat; downbearing qì means cold.
- This formula is a combination of *Guì Zhī Tāng* and *Xiǎo Chái Hú Tāng*, but with *chái hú, guì zhī,* and *dà zǎo* removed. It treats combined tàiyáng and shàoyáng conditions.
- Contraindicated in patients with liver qì disharmony, because the addition of acrid and warm *chuān xiōng* and *dāng guī* causes heat qì to surge upward, and the addition of bitter draining *shēng gé* and *lǐ gēn* fails to treat running piglet.
- The reason why this formula does not include *fú líng* and *guì zhī* even though they are the main medicinals for treating running piglet is that the present indication does not arise from the kidney.

桂枝加桂湯
Guì Zhī Jiā Guì Tāng

guì zhī	桂枝	15g
sháo yào	芍藥	9g
gān cǎo	甘草	6g
shēng jiāng	生薑	9g
dà zǎo	大棗	12 pcs

Indications: Running piglet caused by sweating or hot needling therapy in tàiyáng patterns after sweating.

Analysis:

- A treatment for cold evil erupting as running piglet due to injury to yīn.
- *Guì Zhī Tāng* resolves the external evil.
- The additional *guì zhī* frees the flow of kidney qì.
- The formula exemplifies the rule "Above, protect the fire of shàoyīn; below, warm the water of shàoyīn."

茯苓桂枝甘草大棗湯
Fú Líng Guì Zhī Gān Cǎo Dà Zào Tāng

fú líng	茯苓	24g
gān cǎo	甘草	6g
dà zǎo	大棗	15 pcs
guì zhī	桂枝	12g

Indications: Tàiyáng disease after sweating with palpitations below the navel, which is about to turn into running piglet.

Analysis:

- Treats tàiyáng conditions where sweating has damaged kidney qì.
- *Guì zhī* protects heart qì in the upper body.
- *Fú líng* calms kidney qì in the lower body, hereby transforming water qì in tàiyáng.
- *Gān cǎo* and *dà zǎo* supplement center earth and control the flooding of water evil.

栝蔞薤白白酒湯
Guā Lóu Xiè Bái Bái Jiǔ Tāng

guā lóu shí	栝蔞實	1 pc
xiè bái	薤白	100ml
bái jiǔ	白酒	1,400ml

Indications: Chest impediment, with panting and coughing up spittle, pain in the chest and back, shortness of qì, and a pulse that is sunken and slow at *cùn kǒu* but small, tight, and rapid above *guān*.

Analysis:

- When yīn evil takes up residence in the chest, which is the path of the breath, it stops yáng qì, causing the symptoms described above.
- *Guā lóu* opens the chest bind.
- *Xiè bái* diffuses heart yáng.
- *Bái jiǔ* dissipates impediment and frees yáng, leading it to circulate all throughout the body.

栝蔞薤白半夏湯
Guā Lóu Xiè Bái Bàn Xià Tāng

guā lóu shí	栝蔞實	1 pc
xiè bái	薤白	9g
bàn xià	半夏	100ml
bái jiǔ	白酒	2 liters

Indications: Impediment in the chest with inability to lie down and pain in the heart penetrating to the back.

Analysis:

- This is *Guā Lóu Xiè Bái Bái Jiǔ Tāng* with the addition of *bàn xià*.
- It is able to harmonize the stomach and free the flow of yīn and yáng, in addition to sweeping away rheum.

枳實栝蔞薤白桂枝湯
Zhǐ Shí Guā Lóu Xiè Bái Guì Zhī Tāng

zhǐ shí	枳實	4 pcs
xiè bái	薤白	100ml
guì zhī	桂枝	3g
hòu pò	厚朴	12g
guā lóu shí	栝蔞實	1 pc

Indications: Chest impediment and glomus qì in the heart, with retention and binding in the chest, fullness in the chest, and counterflow below the rib-sides scraping against the heart.

Analysis:

- *Zhǐ shí* and *hòu pò* drain the glomus fullness, move the retention and binding, and downbear the scraping counterflow.
- *Guì zhī* is able to transform the qì of tàiyáng, so that the stagnation and congestion in the chest opens up on its own.
- *Xiè bái* and *guā lóu gēn* are specific medicinals for treating glomus.

人參湯
Rén Shēn Tāng

guì zhī	桂枝	12g
gān cǎo	甘草	12g
rén shēn	人參	9g
gān jiāng	乾薑	9g
bái zhú	白朮	9g

Indications: Tàiyáng disease with the external symptoms still present but complicated by heat and diarrhea, glomus and hardness below the heart, and impediment in the chest.

Analysis:

- Identical with *Guì Zhī Rén Shēn Tāng.*
- In unresolved tàiyáng disease, frequent (and erroneous) treatment with precipitation causes vacuity in the interior, as a result of which the exterior heat is trapped in the interior, forming diarrhea.
- Because chest yáng falls downward and yīn cold rises up, glomus forms.
- *Guì zhī* leads the evil to be outthrust.
- *Gān jiāng* frees the flow of chest yáng and thereby arouses the evil entrapped in the lower body.
- *Bái zhú* secures the spleen and thereby stops the diarrhea complicated by heat.
- *Rén shēn* and *gān cǎo* assist *gān jiāng* and *bái zhú* to support qì, as a result of which chest yáng is able to flow freely and the diarrhea can be checked.
- This formula is a special treatment for vacuity due to glomus and diarrhea by means of sweetness and warmth.

茯苓杏仁甘草湯
Fú Líng Xìng Rén Gān Cǎo Tāng

fú líng	茯苓	9g
xìng rén	杏仁	50 pcs
gān cǎo	甘草	3g

Indications: Impediment in the chest with shortness of breath.

Analysis:

- Treats conditions due to water evil shooting up into the lung and obstructing its emission of qì.
- *Gān cǎo* calms spleen qì.
- *Xìng rén* opens and drains lung qì.
- *Fú líng* clears management and regulation and causes water to flow smoothly down into the lower body, as a result of which the flow of qì regulates itself.
- This formula is comparable in its action to *Jú Pí Zhǐ Shí Shēng Jiāng Tāng*, but uses bland percolation instead of acrid warmth.

橘皮枳實生薑湯
Jú Pí Zhǐ Shí Shēng Jiāng Tāng

jú pí	橘皮	48g
zhǐ shí	枳實	9g
shēng jiāng	生薑	24g

Indications: Impediment in the chest with qì congestion, shortness of breath, a depressed feeling like fullness, choking and itchy scratching, rough dryness in the throat, and foaming at the mouth.

Analysis:

- Treats conditions caused by external evil stirring up internal rheum, which is filling up the highest place and blocking the pathways of qì.
- Warm acrid medicinals are indispensable for sweeping away the rheum and dissipating the evil, hence the formula uses large amounts of greatly acrid and warm *jú pí* and *shēng jiāng*.
- Bitter and discharging medicinals are indispensable for breaking up congestion and balancing qì, hence the formula includes *zhǐ shí*.

薏苡附子散
Yì Yǐ Fù Zǐ Sǎn

yì yǐ rén	薏苡仁	45g
dà fù zǐ	大附子	10 pcs

Indications: Impediment in the chest with laxness and hypertonicity.

Analysis:

- Being endowed with the qì of yángmíng metal, *yì yǐ rén* is able to restrain wind. Since the liver is the organ of wind and rules the sinews, it is able to control the alternating laxness and hypertonicity in the sinews.
- This action is combined with the effect of *fù zǐ* to strongly supplement yáng qì.

桂枝生薑枳實湯
Guì Zhī Shēng Jiāng Zhǐ Shí Tāng

guì zhī	桂枝	9g
shēng jiāng	生薑	9g
zhǐ shí	枳實	15g

Indications: Glomus in the heart, with all forms of counterflow and suspension pain in the heart.

Analysis:

- All these indications are related to heart yáng being vacuous and failing to spread, and to yīn evil lying latent and causing glomus.
- The red color of *guì zhī* supplements the heart and strengthens yáng.
- The acridity of *shēng jiāng* dissipates cold and downbears counterflow.
- The bitter flavor and fragrant qì of *zhǐ shí* guides the acrid warmth of *shēng jiāng* and *guì zhī* to circulate throughout the upper and lower body.

烏頭赤石脂丸
Wū Tóu Chì Shí Zhī Wán

wū tóu	烏頭	0.75g
shǔ jiāo	蜀椒	3g
gān jiāng	乾薑	3g
fù zǐ	附子	1.5g
chì shí zhī	赤石脂	3g

Indications: Heart pain penetrating to the back and back pain penetrating to the heart.

Analysis:

- Anguishing pain that affects both the front and back is a manifestation of disorder in both the qì and blood aspects. If we use only medicinals that treat the qì aspect, we will only further increase the pain and thereby place the patient in grave danger.
- *Shǔ jiāo* and *wū tóu* with their acrid spiciness use warmth to dissipate the yīn evil.
- Because the disordered qì in the chest and back is difficult to calm, the formula includes *gān jiāng* for its guarding effect and *chì shí zhī* for its astringing effect, to fill in the new path of reverse qì surging transversely.

九痛丸
Jiǔ Tòng Wán

fù zǐ	附子	9g
shēng láng yá	生狼牙	3g
bā dòu	巴豆	3g
gān jiāng	乾薑	3g
wú zhū yú	吳茱萸	3g
rén shēn	人參	3g

Indications: The nine forms of heart pain and sudden malignity strike with abdominal distention and inability to speak. Also treats cold that has been accumulating over many years and is now pouring out, manifesting in heart and chest pain. Also treats patterns of surging cold with ascent of qì, falling of a horse or a vehicle, and blood disease.

Analysis:

- "Nine forms of heart pain" is another name for evil in the kidney overcoming the heart and for leg qì rushing against the heart, causing the violent patterns of guest evil.
- This formula uses warm and dissipating medicinals with the addition of *shēng láng yá, bā dòu,* and *wú zhū yú,* to drive the evil out through the yīn orifices.
- Without smashing the nest, you will not be able to dissipate the evil that has seized the chest and formed hard ramparts.

附子粳米湯
Fù Zǐ Jīng Mǐ Tāng

fù zǐ	附子	1 pc
bàn xià	半夏	100ml
jīng mǐ	粳米	100ml
gān cǎo	甘草	3g
dà zǎo	大棗	10 pcs

Indications: Cold qì in the abdomen, with rumbling intestines, slicing pain, counterflow and fullness in the chest and rib-sides, and retching and vomiting.

Analysis:

- *Bàn xià* downbears qì, thereby treating the rumbling intestines, counterflow fullness, and vomiting.
- *Fù zǐ* dispels cold, thereby treating the slicing pain in the abdomen, which is a manifestation of cold.
- These medicinals are assisted by *gān cǎo, jīng mǐ,* and *dà zǎo,* for their ability to harmonize center earth, which is the central point where qì counterflow in the upper body and formation of cold in the lower body intersect.

厚朴七物湯
Hòu Pò Qī Wù Tāng

hòu pò	厚朴	24g
gān cǎo	甘草	9g
dà huáng	大黃	9g
dà zǎo	大棗	10 pcs
zhǐ shí	枳實	5 pcs
guì zhī	桂枝	6g
shēng jiāng	生薑	15g

Indications: Abdominal fullness with heat effusion that has persisted for ten days, a floating and rapid pulse, and eating and drinking as usual.

Analysis:

- Abdominal fullness and a rapid pulse indicate a repletion evil in the interior. Hence this condition has to be treated by dual resolution.
- *Guì Zhī Tāng* without the bitter cold of *sháo yào* resolves the exterior evil and harmonizes construction and defense.
- *Xiǎo Chéng Qì Tāng* sweeps the stomach and intestines to drain interior repletion, since right qì will be unable to recover if the evil is not removed.
- Retching means qì counterflow in the upper body, for which we use *bàn xià* to downbear it.
- The reason why precipitating *dà huáng* is removed is that as long as the exterior evil is not resolved yet, there is a risk that it can double the damage to stomach qì and entrap the evil.
- For predominance of cold, add *shēng jiāng* to dissipate it.

大柴胡湯
Dà Chái Hú Tāng

chái hú	柴胡	24g
huáng qín	黃芩	9g
sháo yào	芍藥	9g
bàn xià	半夏	100ml
zhǐ shí	枳實	4 pcs
dà huáng	大黃	6g
dà zǎo	大棗	12 pcs
shēng jiāng	生薑	15g

Indications: Cold damage that has entered yángmíng without completely leaving shàoyáng, with heart vexation and constipation, hardness and fullness below the chest, incessant retching and vomiting, intermittent cold and heat, and a sunken and replete pulse.

Analysis:

- *Xiǎo Chái Hú* patterns are dominated by intermittent cold and heat in conjunction with fullness below the rib-sides. In patients where the disease has spread to the stomach, we still do not see more than heart vexation and tendency to retching. Even though liver evil has already invaded the stomach, the stomach is not yet greatly affected and shàoyáng signs predominate over yángmíng signs.
- By contrast, the present formula addresses conditions where the patient is suffering from severe intermittent cold and heat, hardness and fullness below the chest, and incessant retching and vomiting, as well as heart vexation and constipation. These symptoms show that the heat binding in the stomach is already severe, hence yángmíng signs predominate over shàoyáng signs.
- In such cases, remove the *rén shēn* and *gān cǎo* from *Xiǎo Chái Hú Tāng* to avoid stagnation.
- The formula uses *chái hú* and *huáng qín* to course shàoyáng as the path on which the evil has arrived, to clear heat.
- *Sháo yào* assists *chái hú* in discharging the liver evil that has invaded the stomach, thereby checking the retching.
- *Bàn xià* harmonizes stagnant stomach qì.
- *Zhǐ shí* and *dà huáng* attack fullness and clear heat.
- *Shēng jiāng* and *dà zǎo* allow stomach qì to recover from its fatigue.
- Hence *Dà Chái Hú Tāng* is a formula to rule conditions where stomach disease is already severe but shàoyáng conditions are not yet eliminated.

厚朴三物湯

Hòu Pò Sān Wù Tāng

hòu pò	厚朴	24g
dà huáng	大黃	12g
zhǐ shí	枳實	5 pcs

Indications: Abdominal fullness and pain with constipation.

Analysis:

- Supporting qì means to sweep away repletion. Hence the sovereign of this formula is *dà huáng*.
- The significance of this formula lies in moving qì, hence the second sovereign is *hòu pò*.
- We do not reduce the amount of *dà huáng* here because you must first free defecation before you can move qì. Free flow of bowel qì means no pain.

大承氣湯

Dà Chéng Qì Tāng

dà huáng	大黃	12g
hòu pò	厚朴	24g
zhǐ shí	枳實	5 pcs
máng xiāo	芒硝	60ml

Indications: Repletion heat in yángmíng, with dry feces hardening and binding in the intestines and fullness and pain in the abdomen.

Analysis:

- Stagnating filth in the intestines is due to qì being unable to move and the fluids being unable to moisten.
- *Dà huáng* here clears the heat; *máng xiāo* moistens the dryness; *hòu pò* moves the qì; *zhǐ shí* attacks hardness.
- This formula is indicated for heat evil that has spread to the interior, which manifests in glomus, fullness, dryness, and repletion and hardness.
- If the exterior evil is not yet resolved or there is hardness and fullness below the heart, or redness in the face, or reduced appetite, or increased retching or a slow pulse or internal exhaustion of the fluids causing reduced urination, any formulas related to *Chéng Qì Tāng* are contraindicated!

大建中湯

Dà Jiàn Zhōng Tāng

shǔ jiāo	蜀椒	40ml
gān jiāng	乾薑	12g
rén shēn	人參	6g

Indications: Being struck by severe cold in the heart or chest, with pain, retching with inability to eat or drink, abdominal fullness surging upward and lifting the skin, appearing like hands or feet, and pain in the upper and lower body so bad that you cannot touch the area around it.

Analysis:

- All these symptoms indicate a severe cold patterns. Hence the formula uses such large amounts of *gān jiāng* as the sovereign, to warm the cold of center earth.
- *Rén shēn* and malt sugar as ministers fortify qì in the center burner.
- Being pure yáng by nature, the assistant *shǔ jiāo* outthrusts the lower body and settles the counterflow of the yīn evil. It also aids *gān jiāng* in arousing the yáng in center earth.
- Drinking down some gruel a short while

after consuming the medicine also warms and nourishes the qì in the center burner.

大黃附子湯

Dà Huáng Fù Zǐ Tāng

dà huáng	大黃	9g
fù zǐ	附子	3 pcs
xì xīn	細辛	6g

Indications: One-sided pain below the rib-side, heat effusion, and a tight and string-like pulse.
Analysis:

- The three *Chéng Qì Tāng* formulas are soft preparations for cold precipitation.
- *Bái Sǎn* and *Bèi Jí Wán* are hard preparations for hot precipitation.
- *Fù Zǐ Xiè Xīn Tāng* and *Dà Huáng Fù Zǐ Tāng* are combination treatments to rescue the patient from cold and heat binding together and hardness and softness relieving each other.
- In this formula, *xì xīn* assists *fù zǐ* in attacking the cold binding below the rib-sides.
- This action is combined with the cold of *dà huáng* to lead it. Thus, cold and heat and the methods of warming and attacking are used together.

赤丸方

Chì Wán Fāng

wū tóu	烏頭	6g
fú líng	茯苓	12g
xì xīn	細辛	3g
bàn xià	半夏	12g

Indications: Cold qì with reversal counterflow.
Analysis:

- Cold qì with reversal counterflow means that yīn evil is exuberant.
- In this formula, *wū tóu* and *xì xīn* to warm and dissipate the exuberant cold.
- *Fú líng* and *bàn xià* downbear and drain the qì ascending counterflow.
- And the color of *zhū shā* has the effect of settling the floating of cold qì and protecting the heart ruler.

大烏頭煎

Dà Wū Tóu Jiān

wū tóu	烏頭	5 large pcs

Indications: Cold mounting with gripping pain in the abdomen, hypertonicity in the five viscera, inability to turn to the side, retracted genitals and reversal in the extremities, possibly abdominal fullness, aversion to cold, and lack of appetite, and a sunken and tight pulse.
Analysis:

- This formula is a treatment for warming the center, strengthening yáng, and strongly breaking up yīn evil.

當歸生薑羊肉湯
Dāng Guī Shēng Jiāng Yáng Ròu Tāng

dāng guī	當歸	9g
shēng jiāng	生薑	15g
yáng ròu	羊肉	48g

Indications: Cold mounting in the abdomen with vacuity taxation and insufficiency. Also treats chronic abdominal pain after childbirth in women.

Analysis:

- Cold mounting should be attacked with warmth, but in patients with vacuity taxation and insufficiency, you cannot attack.
- Abdominal pain should be treated by freeing and discharging, but after childbirth, the vacuity of the body means that you cannot discharge.
- Therefore this method here is designed to free the flow and supplement at the same time, to move blood without damaging blood, and to poke qì without exhausting qì.
- In this formula, *dāng guī* relieves pain by moving stagnation in the blood aspect while *shēng jiāng* relieves pain by diffusing stagnation in the qì aspect.
- The rich thick nature of mutton enriches and supplements.

烏頭桂枝湯
Wū Tóu Guì Zhī Tāng

wū tóu	烏頭	5 pcs
mì	蜜	96g
guì zhī tāng	桂枝湯	100ml

Indications: Cold mounting with pain in the center of the abdomen, counterflow cold, and numbness in the hands and feet.

柴胡桂枝湯
Chái Hú Guì Zhī Tāng

chái hú	柴胡	12g
huáng qín	黃芩	4.5g
rén shēn	人參	4.5g
bàn xià	半夏	50ml
dà zǎo	大棗	12 pcs
shēng jiāng	生薑	9g
gān cǎo	甘草	3g
guì zhī	桂枝	4.5g
sháo yào	芍藥	4.5g

Indications: Cold damage with heat effusion, slight aversion to cold, soreness and vexation in the joints of the extremities, mild retching, propping binding below the heart, unresolved external symptoms, possibly profuse sweating, yáng collapse with delirious raving, possibly sudden pain in the heart and abdomen.

Analysis:

- This formula is a combination of *Xiǎo Chái Hú Tāng* and *Guì Zhī Tāng* to treat combined shàoyáng and tàiyáng disease.
- *Guì Zhī Tāng* resolves the fleshy exterior of tàiyáng and moreover balances the fleshy exterior of all the channels.
- *Xiǎo Chái Hú Tāng* resolves the half exterior of shàoyáng and also harmonizes the half exterior of the three yáng channels.
- On the sixth or seventh day of cold damage disorders, the patient has passed through a complete cycle. If you still see the exterior

signs of heat effusion and aversion to cold and in addition see the interior signs of propping binding below the heart, you must adopt the method of resolving both the interior and exterior.

- Hence use the half of *Guì Zhī Tāng* to dissipate the evil that is not completely eliminated in tàiyáng, and use the half of *Xiǎo Chái Hú Tāng* to resolve the mild binding in shàoyáng.
- This is Zhāng Zhòngjǐng's method for a mild preparation for dual resolution.

走馬湯

Zǒu Mǎ Tāng

bā dòu	巴豆	2 pcs
xìng rén	杏仁	2 pcs

Indications: Flying corpse, being hit by demons, malignity strike, with heart pain, abdominal distention, and stopped defecation.

Analysis:

- Malignity strike with heart pain and stopped defecation indicates repletion evil.
- In the formula, *bā dòu* is warm and acrid and highly toxic. It eliminates demonic infixation and *gǔ* poisoning. It also pierces the pathways of water and grain.
- *Xìng rén* is sweet, bitter, and warm, and mildly toxic. It enters the lung channel. Since malignity and poisons enter through the mouth and nose, they should also be attacked from the highest origin of the skin and body hair.
- Contraindicated in patients with vacuity! It is only for conditions with cold repletion and greatly toxic evil qì.

Texts

People

Medicinals

Formulas

Indications

A

B

C

D

金匱方歌括

E

F

金匱方歌括

I

J

K

Y

The Chinese Medicine Database

www.cm-db.com

The Chinese Medicine Database has been organized around one central principle -- translation of Classical Chinese texts, and dissemination of that information.

There are thousands of Chinese medicine texts that have never been translated. We have compiled a small list on our website of the ones that we have found, but we believe that there are tens of thousands of documents that span from pre-Republican times to the Han dynasty. Most of these documents will never be read by people in the West, simply because of lack of translation.

We have created a vehicle, that allows interested practitioners, students, institutions, and scholars to help support and fund the translation of these documents, and then mine and synthesize the data that is gained from these texts.

The Database contains:

Monographs on:

- 673 Single Herbs
- 1485 Formulas
- Mayway's Patents
- ITM's Formulations
- Golden Flowers Formulations
- Health Concerns Formulations
- Blue Poppy's Patents
- Classical Pearls Formulations by Heiner Fruehauf
- OBGYN Modifications to Formulas
- Single Points: the 361 Regular Points

15,000 Western Diagnoses with ICD-9 Codes

A Chinese-English dictionary:

Containing over 100,000 terms, including the Eastland and the WHO term sets.

A Western Book search containing:

- Fenners Complete Formulary
  - by B. Fenner
- The 1918 Dispensatory of the United States of America
  - Edited by Joseph P. Remington, Horatio C. Woods and others
- The Eclectic Materia Medica, Pharmacology and Therapeutics
  - by Harvey Wickes Felter, M.D.

A Personal Dashboard, which allows users to:

- Blog
- Take notes on any monograph.
- Search for other users by city, state, country and name.
- Make friends all around the world.

Share and compare notes with friends.
Personalize your dashboard by adding photos, and information about your practice.

Translations:

Shāng Hán Lái Sū Jí 傷寒來蘇集: Renewal of Treatise on Cold Damage
Qí Jīng Bā Mài Kǎo 奇經八脈考: Explanation of the Eight Vessels of the Marvellous Meridians
Shāng Hán Míng Lǐ Lùn 傷寒明理論: Treatise on Enlightening the Principles of Cold Damage.
Wú Jū Tōng Yī àn 吴鞠通医案: Case Studies of Wú Jū-tōng
The Nán Jīng 難經: The Classic of Difficulties
The Zang Fu Biao Ben Han Re Xu Shi Yong Yao Shi 臟腑標本寒熱虛實用藥式: Viscera and Bowels, Tip and Root, Cold and Heat, Vacuity and Repletion Model for Using Medicinals
Bèi Jí Qiān Jīn Yào Fāng 備急千金要方: Essential Prescriptions Worth a Thousand Gold Pieces For Emergencies. vol. 2-4
Wēn Rè Lún 温熱論: Treatise on Warm Heat Disease
Shāng Hán Shé Jiàn 傷寒舌鑒: Tongue Mirror of Cold Damage
Xǔ Shì Yī àn 許氏醫案: Case Histories of Master Xu
Fǔ Xìng Jué Zāng Fǔ Yòng Yào Fǎ Yào 輔行決臟腑用藥法要: Secret Instructions for Assisting the Body: Essential Methods for the Application of Drugs to the Viscera & Bowels
Biāo Yōu Fù (annotation) 標幽賦（ 楊氏註解 ）: Indicating the Obscure
Liú Juān Zǐ Guǐ Yí Fāng 劉涓子鬼遺方: Liu Juanzi's Formulas Inherited from Ghosts
Shèn Jí Chú Yán 慎疾芻言: Precautions in Illness: My Humble Thoughts
Yào Zhèng Jì Yí 藥症忌宜: Medicinals & Patterns Contraindications & Appropriate [Choices]

Benefits:

Subscribers to the Database receive a 10% discount on our published books when they are in pre-release.

We translate texts as often, and in quantities that reflect our user base. The larger amount of subscribers that we have, the more translation that we can accomplish.

Published Books:

2008 Bèi Jí Qiān Jīn Yào Fāng 備急千金要方: Essential Prescriptions Worth a Thousand Gold Pieces For Emergencies. vol. 2-4 by Sūn Sī Miǎo 孫思邈
Translated by Sabine Wilms.
ISBN 978-0-9799552-0-4

2010 Zhēn Jiǔ Dà Chéng 針灸大成: The Great Compendium of Acupuncture & Moxabustion vol. I by Yáng Jì Zhōu 楊繼州
Translated by Sabine Wilms.
ISBN 978-0-9799552-2-8

2010 Zhēn Jiǔ Dà Chéng 針灸大成: The Great Compendium of Acupuncture & Moxabustion vol. V by Yáng Jì Zhōu 楊繼州
Translated by Lorraine Wilcox.
ISBN 978-0-9799552-4-2

www.ingramcontent.com/pod-product-compliance
Lightning Source LLC
LaVergne TN
LVHW080642011026
849160LV00014B/1297